Superbly Natural Surgery

One Woman's Experience in The Philippines

To Gmma

Love

Theresa

Theresa Jones

Published by Paragon Publishing

© Theresa Jones 2021

superblynaturalsurgery@gmail.com

ISBN 978-1-78222-844-8

Book design, layout and production management by Into Print
www.intoprint.net, +44 (0)1604 832140

With appreciation I dedicate this book to

Grayle for his understanding and for allowing me to be me
and giving me the space;
and to Ross for his understanding and support

One Woman's Experience

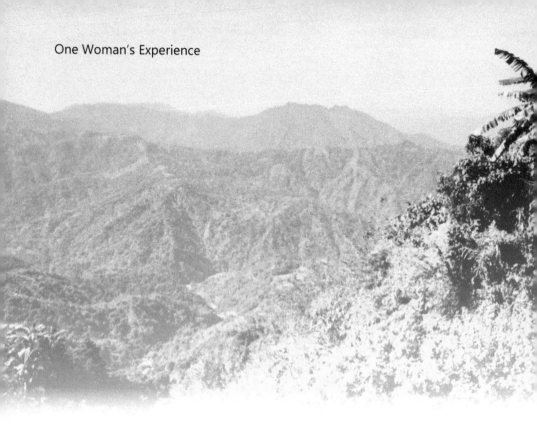

FOREWORD

This book was never meant to be, but ...

I wrote the basis of this book about three years ago, not necessarily with a view to having it published, more an exercise in book writing, and it is an interesting story and it is a true story. It is also an intimate story and for this reason, I have changed the names of the characters and anything which may identify them because at the time, we agreed to not share this information.

Once I had written the outline, I was able to contact the person I refer to as Paul to ask if he would mind me publishing and he said he felt comfortable with that so long as I did not identify him or the group. I no longer have contact details for the others and feel it fair to assume that their response would be similar. However, the man I refer to as Roger, was Roger who, I understand, passed away in around 2015 and I feel that he should be recognised and acknowledged for the amazing work he was here on Earth to do. He was a special man with many gifts using frequency and vibration.

In the last few weeks I have felt a real sense of urgency to share this information because recently I learned of a new technology in medicine, a technology using frequency to heal people in the most amazing ways and I understand it is just a matter of divine timing before this will be available worldwide. I quote:

"These Quantum Therapy Med-Beds will come in three different varieties and three unique functions; they all work on various vibrational and frequency levels with refracting lenses and 3D scanners, as well as surgically precise lasers for opening and closing wounds."

These high frequency beds are capable of producing results of which we could only ever have dreamed. The results will be stunning and I feel that my story may bring some enlightenment and visual awakening of what is possible, that anything is possible, if we are open to possibilities. Because the work Roger was doing using only frequency and vibration, and therefore perhaps in alignment with these Med-Beds, that the time to publish this book, if ever I was going to, was now.

In this time of isolation and disconnection from the world, being contained and not distracted, I had been guided to bring this book back from its dormancy in the hope that it may contribute in some small way to the conscious awakening of humanity. This particular time in history that we are living through, right now, is **biblical** and we are seeing the most major shift in human consciousness. The vibration of the planet is being raised, and I believe we will be living in a more spiritual world, a kinder world, a world in which we will wish to be of service to others and feel wonderful about doing so. I feel lucky to be alive at this time to experience what is happening and what is about to happen.

March 2021

Theresa

superblynaturalsurgery@gmail.com

Chapter 1

The Epiphany

I had told few people my story, never all of it, but with those I did share, women found it fascinating; men ran for the hills, holding their groins.

The clock on the kitchen wall showed five to six. It was a Tuesday afternoon towards the end of October 2001, the dark winter night was settling in. I had driven home from my hospital appointment in Winchester, with the words of the consultant bounding around inside my head. "For three months, pretty much, you will be confined to the house, unable to lift anything more than a cup of tea, no driving, nothing strenuous, reliant on others ..." The words kept bombarding me. Such thoughts were truly alarming and already I was feeling the sense of being trapped, trapped inside my house, my home, much of my independence denied, not wanting to be a burden, yet would be so, and, I would be alone for much of the day. The depression I was anticipating was already permeating within me.

How could I sentence myself to this term of confinement and dependency? I was well, in good health, not in pain. This did not sit well with me and I didn't believe it had to be this way, it didn't feel congruent with who I was. I was a free spirit who had spent many years learning to look after my own health, using natural remedies such as homeopathy, osteopathy, and in more recent years an amazing Applied Kineisiologist whose practice covered all of these disciplines plus the mental and emotional body. So I knew that mainstream medicine was not the only answer, there would be an alternative and I also knew that I had choice. The consultant had simply given his advice and his opinion which I could choose to take, or leave, or find an alternative idea. There had to be another way, but at that exact precise moment I did not know what that way was. I had decided to sit with it as I drove back home.

My son was in the kitchen when I arrived, and as I looked at the clock I explained to him that the consultant had suggested that my fist-sized fibroid and cyst on my ovary be surgically removed and that would mean me being reliant on him and my husband for a good part of three months, or, I could ignore it and hope nothing negative would happen. That would be an easy way but something about that felt a little out of kilter.

But, as I was imparting this to him, I suddenly had an epiphany, a light-bulb moment. It came to me in a flash. There was, possibly, another option. From deep within my recall, I remembered an article I had seen some two years earlier and had sent for the full details, never thinking for a moment I would have the need to be involved, although clearly I had been interested and my curiosity piqued.

A daytime television magazine programme had featured a guy involved in natural healing, and I had been intrigued, the concept so absolutely resonating with me, never occurring to me that this maybe was not real, would not work. I had sent for the information and then had filed it away somewhere, "just in case", but where? I stood still, grounded myself and allowed my mind to drift into emptiness. Almost instantly, I felt myself drawn to a box-file which I had recently, for some odd reason, placed on the sideboard in the dining room. I raised the lid, and there, looking right at me, sitting on top of all the other papers, was the article. I lifted it from the box, held it to my chest, and looked skywards with thanks of appreciation and gratitude.

Clutching it firmly in my hand, I sprang up the flight of stairs to my studio, picked up the landline phone and dialled the number at the bottom of the page. A man answered.

"Would that be Paul?" I asked.

"Yes," a foreign sounding voice answered.

"Hello Paul, you sent me your article a couple of years back. I have just been advised by my consultant to have surgery, I don't wish to take his advice, and am looking for an alternative, and what you are offering feels very congruent to me, and I am wondering if you will be organising another trip any time soon?"

"Actually," he responded, "Yes, there is one organised and we will be leaving in three weeks' time and there happens to be just one space left if you would like it, and, so long as you are suitable. You will need to attend an interview with me before we leave, but you are welcome to join us. I will send you the details of the flights you will need to organise. What is your email address and I will do that right now?"

I heard myself giving Paul my contact details, thanked him profusely and put down the phone. I stood and stared blankly into the room. My goodness, I couldn't quite believe what I had just asked for, and agreed to, and it took me some moments for that to integrate and process. And then, when the realisation hit me, my mood changed dramatically, and I bounded back down the stairs to share my news. I was bubbling. I had found an alternative way of dealing with my issue, and, in the process, would have an adventure. How does life get any better than this, I thought?

I arrived in the hall-way, just as my husband arrived home and had walked into the kitchen where my son was making coffee. They could both see that I had something to share with them, and they both stood and looked at me expectantly. I quickly and animatedly explained the advice the consultant had given me and that I couldn't bear the thought of three months trapped and dependent on them. It wasn't fair any of us and that I had found an alternative solution. I announced my plans. They both looked at me with some bemusement and intrigue.

In The Philippines was a psychic bare-hand surgeon who carried out surgery without anaesthetic, without pain, with no side effects, and virtually no healing time and Paul occasionally took small groups to him for healing and that I had spoken with him and I could join them on the next trip, in three weeks' time. All credit to them, they did not suggest I was crazy but began asking lots of questions, some of which I could answer, most of which I couldn't, but I felt they understood my reasoning.

In the midst of the questioning, and for some reason unbeknown to me, I had found myself glancing at the clock again. I did a double take. "Surely not, it can't only be six o'clock? How could that be? I had only arrived home five minutes before, yet I had done so much in that short time span?" I reasoned with myself that I must have briefly slipped into a time warp that had allowed me to achieve so much. I felt that was a really good omen; it had a good energy about it and confirmed to me that I was definitely on the right path, and my intuition was serving me well.

Instinctively, I knew I would be "suitable" for the trip. Paul forwarded the information I would need as soon as we had finished our conversation, and I went ahead and called the airline. I was somewhat relieved to be able to book the same flight as the group with United Emirates, from London Heathrow to Manila, in The Philippines. I called Paul to confirm that I had arranged my flight, and then arranged to visit him one evening of the following week, as he had asked.

Both my husband and I visited Paul for my compulsory interview. Paul had to be sure I was doing the right thing for me, and that I had no hang-ups or misconceptions, and that I had a complete understanding and acceptance of what to expect. Also he needed to feel that I would gel with the rest of the group! It was important that we were all singing from the same song sheet, and that our intentions were clear. All was well, I had passed my interview and was accepted on the trip.

I was excited. Just a fortnight to go, and I would be off on a once in a lifetime adventure which would restore my body to a healthy being.

Chapter 2

New Friends at Heathrow

It was November, one of those wintry cold but bright afternoons, as we pulled up at the drop-off point at Heathrow Airport. My husband unloaded my suitcase from the car and lowered the boot. We turned and faced each other, knowing that we would be apart for ten days. We hugged a deep hug and kissed. I knew he was feeling more than a little anxious, more than a little sad and more than a little envious as he stepped back into the car. He turned to me, waved and drove off, very slowly. I really felt for him in that moment. He had not tried to stop me from going, or tried to make me feel guilty, or complained about the cost, nothing, and I so appreciated and loved him for that. But this was something I needed to do for myself. This was part of my journey, an important part, and at that moment, I had no way of knowing just how important.

I held that moment, tinged with my own sadness and a very full heart, and watched the car as it slowly disappeared down the rank towards the main airport road and out of sight. I took a deep breath and grabbed my case.

I turned and headed through the automatic doors of the terminal building, to be greeted by a toddler running fearlessly towards me. Instinctively, I let go of my case and reached down and grabbed him by the arm and held him as his mother, desperately calling his name, trailed behind him with an arm outstretched. Full of apology and gratitude, she took him from me and they both disappeared back into the crowd.

The airport was heaving with activity, jam-packed full of families struggling with both their luggage trollies and impatient offspring, whilst trying to locate their particular check-in desks. I loved it, it was exciting and I felt particularly energised. My mood had changed.

It wouldn't be long before I would be meeting my fellow travellers for the very first time. I battled my way through the crowds, trying to find the UAE check-in desks. Once located, I joined the tail-end of one of the queues, all very long and barely moving and I began to feel myself becoming impatient, and a little anxious, as it was feeling important for me to connect with my group before boarding the plane. After all, I was about to embark on an interesting and exciting adventure, and I really didn't want it to get off to a difficult start.

Eventually, with boarding pass in hand, and my suitcase safely deposited with the baggage handlers, I headed off to find my soon-to-be new friends. People were standing around, luggage tucked between their legs, waiting for a seat to become available. Then, at the farthest point, I spotted him. Paul was standing at the end of a row of seats, scanning the crowds back and forth. He saw me coming and smiled, waving a welcoming arm. I could see that the others had already arrived and settled themselves in one of the rows and were making cursory conversation.

"Hi Paul", I called, as I drew closer to him, "am I glad to find you? How are you?"

"Hi", he said, "I am glad you made it and happy you are joining us. Let me introduce you to the rest of the group". He turned to them and they were all looking up at me.

"Allow me introduce you all. This is Theresa, she lives in

Hampshire" he said, looking at them all, and to me he said "This is Ellen and Greg, they are married and this is Andrew and Hannah, and they too are married". We greeted each other taking it in turns to shake hands.

Ellen and Greg, an older couple, retired probably, oozed elegance and style. Ellen, an attractive greying blonde with a good figure and her husband slightly taller than her, a little thick around the middle, balding, and sporting quite a tan. From their accents, they weren't British. Andrew and Hannah were younger, probably in their early to mid-forties with middle class English accents. Andrew, tall and slim, was a good looking man, with short dark wavy hair, whilst his wife was much shorter with a happy freckled face and similar hair type. With the little I knew of Paul and with my own story, we must be, I thought, be a slightly off the wall bunch of individuals.

Once through Passport Control and by way of making conversation, I mentioned to Paul that I had bought chocolate should there be nothing decent when we landed. He barely looked at me as he said that it was not a good idea to take it with me as I would not be allowed to eat it, when we arrived! Really, I thought, really! And that would be because ...?

My disappointment was soon morphed into anxiety. Through the entrance to our waiting area, came a guard with a sniffer dog. Instinctively, the room went very still. The dog walked slowly, sniffing between the rows of seated people. Even though I was perfectly innocent, as I am sure we all were, my heart was beating faster, whilst at the same time I tried to reason with myself how silly, how ridiculous that was. In recent times, there had been many incidents of drug trafficking and the sniffer dogs had become normal procedure at all airports and was particularly stringent in the London airports. But that did not put paid to my angst until, satisfied that we were all innocent and drug-free, the dog turned with its handler and exited the area. The sense of relief was tangible and we all breathed again.

Inside the aircraft, a Boeing 747, we were seated randomly throughout the plane. The others were nowhere to be seen, although I could see Paul some rows behind. We settled ourselves for the long haul ahead.

Chapter 3

The Energy of Money

For almost all the seven hours, I had been sitting in the plane, passing time with food, drinks, movies, reading and the odd nap. I should have felt intrusive when I found myself absorbed watching the Arabs get down onto their knees and pray to Mecca, honouring their religion with spiritual union wherever they were in the world, and totally oblivious to any interested and curious onlookers, such as me.

It was such a relief to be breaking the journey at Dubai Airport to stretch legs and to absorb a totally different reality and culture for a few hours. Paul and I exited the plane at much the same time, and used the travellator which glided us into another world.

Palm trees planted and spectacularly decorated with deep bands of gold hugging the trunks were hit by the sunlight pouring through the high glass ceilings and walls. Light sparkled and spangled the glamour and opulence of this land.

"Come on", said Paul, "Let's go and find the private lounge and eat some local cuisine. We have plenty of time on our hands". We did just that and enjoyed chatting and getting to know a little more about each other's history and future hopes.

Paul expanded more about his work which involved much more than organising these trips. His home, I had noticed, was quite large, although when we had met, I had only seen the sitting room used by his family. However, he explained that he had a large room with adjoining facilities from which he ran courses and his own private practice offering alternative therapies. He regularly held classes teaching Anatomy and Physiology, Reiki, Emotional Freedom Technique, Ear Candling, Face Reading and other such modalities, but his real strength and love was nutrition, and he was devoted to that.

Paul went on to explain that he had had a serious number of cancerous liver tumours and had been determined to heal from them naturally, rather than using western medicine. He had studied and researched, and tried and tested many therapies, and gradually he was almost healed. Part of the healing came through diet, liver cleansing procedures and with the help of the man we were about to visit.

For myself, I recounted a little of my own recent story, that I had had three children, but had very sadly lost two of them. In 1976 our first daughter Kelly had died at less than a month old, without obvious reason. In 1999 and just two and a half years before that trip, we had devastatingly lost our second daughter Laura, suddenly, aged 19, again with no obvious reason. Very fortunately, and thank God, we did still have our son Ross, our middle child. Losing his sister, and us our daughter, had obviously brought us all indescribable amounts of heartache, and pain, and loss, leaving a huge void, which we were all dealing with in our own different ways, always trying to support each other, but often ending failing dismally. We were so lucky, and so very grateful to have lived in a village for more than twenty years, and the villagers positively allowed and encouraged us to use them as a crutch whenever we needed to do so. And so, very appreciatively we did, and often!

Continuing, I expanded that for me, my own true spiritual journey, accessing my own consciousness, really began, the day

Laura died and she connected with all of us. I saw her shadowiness, plasma in a mirror, we all felt her energy, we all knew that she was still close, and as I write this, she still communicates with me most days. This is a true blessing, the knowing that life continues after life.

Feeling comfortable in each other's company we ventured back into the crowds. The energy was tangible, inspirational and vital, filling me with an exhilarating sense of possibility. This was not about being materialistic, but about the energy that money affords us. I was surrounded with abundance, the energy of money, the energy of choice.

Chapter 4

Treasured Memory

Finally, we landed in Manila. It was early evening, dark and there was a chill in the air as we piled into a minibus. Paul had warned us of the dangers of Manila at night, and that we should stay as a group and not to wander off alone. The hotel, at which we would be staying for this one night, was just a short distance, and not in a particularly salubrious area; pavements and shop doorways already were scattered with bodies lying beneath cardboard.

I had stayed at better places, but this would serve me well for a single night, I thought. The flights had been long, and we were all tired and hungry and soon eating at a local restaurant. As much as I would have loved us to explore city life together, to do so at night would have been dangerous, and sleep was beckoning.

Early next morning saw us returning to Manila airport for the final leg of our journey to Baguio, a short flight north of Manila. We had been waiting in the departure lounge. Outside the temperature was already quite warm and we were glad to be out of the sun. An air stewardess arrived and asked us to follow her and we walked across the airfield. There were just a dozen of us headed towards a tiny twin-engine propeller plane, boasting white livery with red Asian Spirit insignia. I felt some excited tension. This plane was small. A couple of men loaded our luggage into the tailpiece. A single metal tread had been lowered from the cabin and one by one we stepped aboard, with our only option being to turn left. Just six rows of seats packed the tiny cabin, 2 seats either side of the aisle. Paul and I found ourselves sitting together - he next to the window and me the aisle. All felt rather cosy and intimate.

The Pilot was within touching distance of his passengers, just a simple plastic sliding window like that of a taxi, between him and us. I could have shaken hands with him, without moving an inch. In the cockpit, he alternated between turning to us with some friendly chat, running through routine procedure with the men on the runway, and taking instructions from Traffic Control. With luggage safely stowed, the stewardess stepped aboard with her back to the pilot; the thickness of a sheet of plastic separating them. She was petite, wearing a scarlet red uniform with a pencil knee-length skirt and fitted jacket, a buttoned white blouse and red stilettos. Her long glossy black hair was swept high on top of her head, beneath a red pill-box hat, make-up immaculately applied. Wearing red lipstick and manicured, painted red nails, she was stunningly beautiful. She held my attention.

The wings of the plane spanned above the height of the windows, and as the engines began to rev, the propellers slowly beginning to turn. The pilot closed the little plastic screen between us, and the stewardess took her cue. In both English and Filipino, she began the compulsory inflight safety routine with some serious professionalism. In both hands, she held up for all of us to see, a shiny safety instruction sheet, and then a lifejacket which she proceeded to demonstrate its use and how it should be worn in the event that things did not pan out as planned. We all sat most attentively, giving her the time and respect she deserved ... until, with both her arms and hands fully extended, she pointed down to the blue lighting system on the floor which would help guide us pass the few seats and then with both arms still pointing forward, she raised them and pointed her hands 90 degrees to her right, indicating where we would find the exit door.

The absolute absurdity of this scene, in this tiny little plane, totally appealed to my sense of humour. Desperately, trying to stifle a stomach-full of giggles, I glanced sideways to Paul. Tears were rolling down his cheeks and he was clasping his body with both arms trying to keep still. Feeling awkward and embarrassed, and trying to be invisible, I looked at the other passengers beside me. They sat, expressionless, po-faced, and not the least bit amused. That was all it took. For me, all sense of propriety was totally lost, and I rocked. She smiled sweetly at each of us, took three strides forward, turned and stepped off the plane, folded the step into the cabin, said goodbye, and shut the door behind her! She had just left us! Our stewardess has jumped off the plane and left us! This completely sent me over the edge again, and has left me with a wonderfully disgraceful memory I will always treasure.

Taxiing the runway, the two little engines roared into life, and in no time at all, we were above the steep and rugged mountainous terrain of Luzon. The richly abundant and verdant green valleys below were peppered with little coloured roof tops and shiny, sparkling ribbons of rivers, snaking their way towards the coast and the South China Sea. It was spectacular to see the geography from such a low altitude and to be able to make out the finer details of the landscape beneath us, not possible in a larger aircraft.

We had been in the air for an hour or so when the plane banked eastwards and into view came the small runway of Loakan Airport, raised above a small purpose built plateau and surrounded by mountains on three sides. It looked a little scary and there seemed little room for pilot error. As the plane descended as we approached the runway, we could see just how densely populated parts of the valley were, and how fragile some of the buildings must be. And then there was a bump as the wheels of the plane touched the runway, and with the full force of applied brakes, gradually came to a halt. As one, it seemed, we all breathed a huge and involuntary thankful sigh of relief. From the outside, somebody opened the door and pulled down the tread. We each gathered our travel bags, stepped down onto the concrete, breathing in the cooler air of the mountain.

The "Asian Spirit"; tiny twin-engine propellor plane

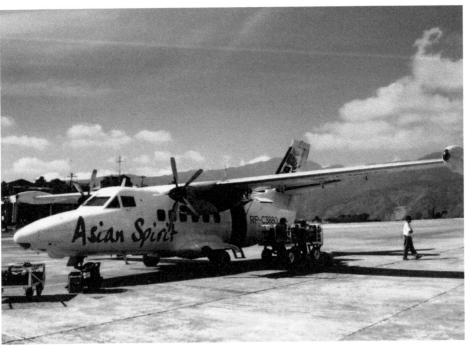

Chapter 5

The Hotel

Excitement was beginning to stir within, my heart dancing a little dance, the next stage of my journey about to unfold. I was here to meet a very special man, perhaps today but Paul needed to have a conversation with him a little later.

The hotel in Baguio had arranged for a minibus to transfer us from the airport to the hotel. It was situated on the main road, nothing special, just basic facilities, clean and utilitarian with an en-suite bathroom. I was grateful my room was at the rear of the building, much quieter than the front. Looking out of the window I was curious about the view. One would assume that any hotel would have been trying to create an attractive ambience with a sense of well-being for its visitors. But here, there was an unexpected and inexplicably strange mix of vistas. Directly below and backing onto the hotel premises, some kind of indeterminable yard used for storing construction materials. Rows of dark wooden office buildings, beneath multi-coloured corrugated tin roofs served the yard. I watched as open backed trucks kept a steady schedule of delivering or collecting materials. It seemed such a strange business activity for an hotel to have associations with and I was thankful that I would not be spending much time there.

But, when I lifted my awareness upwards and away from the ugliness, the view changed dramatically. Looking beyond, stood a magnificent nine storeyed white apartment block, with arched windows and balconies on all elevations, beneath terracotta tiled pyramid roofs and surrounded by amazing sculptural pine trees. Further away and lower down the hill, neighbouring properties were smaller, simpler white apartment buildings and detached white houses, all separated with tall pine trees and small parks. In the very far distance, towering above the roof-tops was the Cordilleras mountain range, protecting those who lived within its boundaries.

Downstairs we all met, murmuring about food and needing to eat. Paul was ahead of us and suggested a café a few doors away for a quick snack before heading into the city.

"This sounds as though it is going to be a long day for us" I said to Paul. "Will we not go to Green Valley today then?"

"Apparently, it would be better to begin tomorrow, fully rested, to gain the most benefit and that makes perfect sense and feels right. So enjoy the day and get a sense of your surroundings and local colour and the vibration of life here".

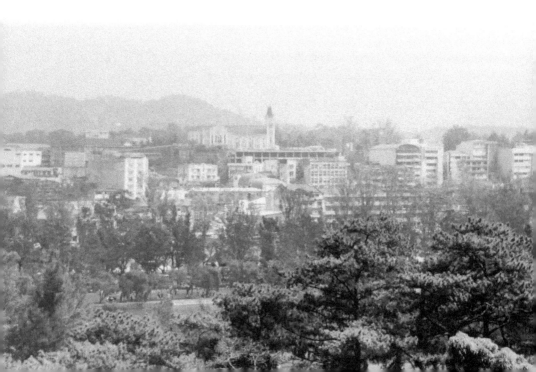

Chapter 6

Baguio and all its Glory

The smells hit us immediately. Concoctions of spices, fruit, meat and fish found its way into our nostrils. The place was fizzing, alive with conversation between traders shouting across the stalls to each other, and customers haggling with stall holders. Steam and smoke rose up from woks sizzling with fish and vegetables to satisfy the hungry hoards. Dogs sniffed their way around the various waste bins, cocking their legs often, as dogs do, and the many cats kept themselves out of harm's way, by leaping up into any secret nook or cranny they could find.

Amidst all the noise and hustle and bustle, and almost unnoticed, a svelte black cat sprang down from the dark and flimsy wooden rafters overhead. Its landing stage was a pile of red plastic crates stacked against the wall by the fish-seller who was sitting on his haunches, bartering with a potential customer. For many moments the cat sat perfectly still. It was eyeing the fish displayed in open crates standing on the grey, uneven and cracked concrete floor. The cat bided its time, it waited, and waited some more, and then, in a single movement, jumped onto the rim of a crate, snatched a fish and scurried away between the feet of the crowd. This was Baguio Market, in all its glory.

The market place itself was widely sprawled, both in the main building and traversing the streets outside. The central block within the main building was built of brick with a traditional roof, but the area had been extended dramatically with simple wooden beams and rafters, topped with coloured corrugated plastic sheets. Strangely, the interior of the market was created into small, tall rooms constructed with wire mesh sheets and filled with dirty cardboard boxes and pallets. This provided alleyways for extra trading areas and allowed sellers to stack all types of potatoes onto the concrete and together with their vital scales propped onto stools and recycled old plastic carrier bags stuffed beneath, they were set. Every inch of trading space was filled. This was (and is) the way of life for many Filipinos.

Staying together as a group was not easy as we drifted amongst and between the vast mazes of stalls, stopping to discover something interesting which fascinated us. Jostling with the crowds, mostly dressed in jeans and tee shirts or anoraks, the hubbub was constant, and I loved watching, listening and observing the people and their way of life, a way quite different from my own. Sometimes I would ask the stall-holder if I may take a photograph, but more often it was a general view that captured my interest. The bright colours of the fruits, or the bare light bulbs strung between the stalls, dangerously hot, or beautifully presented fish, or the hundreds of electricity or telephone cables attached to a single pole.

Clusters of fruit and vegetable stalls were dispersed throughout the whole market, enticing us to buy their super fresh fruit and vegetables, grown locally. Each stall seemed to specialise in just a few vegetables, or just a few fruit. The variety was enormous. Individual stall holders displayed plastic crates of bananas, guavas, papayas, pineapple, kalamansi and coconuts. Vegetables included napa cabbage, water spinach, Chinese cabbage, aubergines, yard long beans, potatoes, carrots, purple yam and sweet potatoes amongst others. Many I recognised, but not all.

The sweet smell of papaya and passion fruit filled the air. Most of the vegetables had already sold out as it was late in the day.

As we continued to drift, we discovered an area dedicated to sausages, amazingly beautifully displayed. Along one wall, traders hired regular small booths, with counter space and metal hanging rails above. Row upon row of pink and brown sausages of all shapes, sizes and flavours hung symmetrically, out and beyond the confines of their own booths, each with the stall holder's name and specialism proudly displayed both above and below the counter.

Filipinos in general do not enjoy a rich economy. Their simple lifestyle forces them to create the best of each situation. These people took their fish to market in simple plastic storage boxes and together with a small folding stool, their market stall was set. They sat in a long line, low on their stools, wearing the seemingly uniform jeans and anorak, often with a woolly hat and flip-flops.

Below left: Fish Market
Below: Baguio Indoor Market

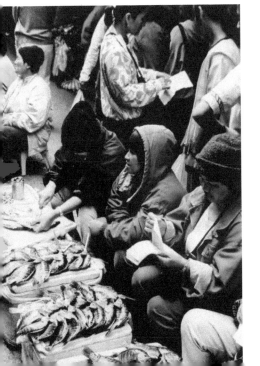 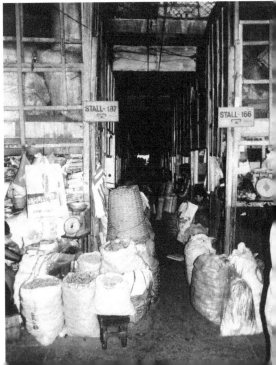

Between the different varieties of fish each person had brought, other traders set up with a few jars of honey, fresh olives or maybe some cabbages; a curious collection.

Men and women juggled the spaces available. Fabrics, were piled high onto make-shift shelving, rolls of natural cottons, modern polyester and threads, stood lined up against the walls. Old broom handles suspended between roof joists made rails to hang jackets and trousers.

Unbelievably, we had spent a couple of hours trawling through alleyways, twists and turns, discovering and getting to know a little of life, and how people lived, up there in the mountains. We found ourselves out in a street with more market, but what struck me particularly, was as far as the eye could see, the quantity of cables strung, in their hundreds, from telegraph pole to telegraph pole, from shop to shop, and apartment to apartment; an organised yet chaotic system keeping the community in touch with each other and the rest of the world.

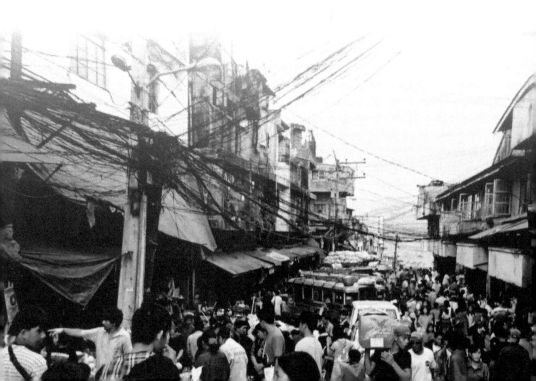

We had had a good taste of this huge market, and now I was ready for a change of pace to explore and discover the city itself.

Baguio City, often referred to as the City of Pines, because of the abundance of pine trees, or, Summer Capital of The Philippines because the Filipinos themselves would often spend their summer holidays there for the relief it brought from the intense heat of the lowlands, usually eight degrees less, somewhere between 15-23 degrees centigrade.

Protected by the sprawling Cordilleras mountain range, Baguio City nestles on a plateau 1,500 feet above sea level, is highly urbanised with uneven hilly terrain and is a puzzling attraction. It is thought that the landscape is still in its infancy with its enduring and natural process of erosion and earthquakes being the cause of its steep ruggedness.

Typical of many tourists when they travel abroad, I couldn't resist the urge to check out property prices and was interested to see that when advertising properties, details not only include those of the actual buildings, but also states the degree of the slope of the terrain, and identify whether it is gently rolling or rugged landscape, and the width of the road frontage.

The day had been long and we were seriously famished so took a taxi to the well-known and recommended Café By The Ruins. It was early evening, with a nip in the air and the sun had slipped slowly away. A wooden pathway margined with boulders and tall jewel coloured vegetation drew us into what appeared to be a cave. Yet crossing the threshold revealed half the ceiling covered in clear plastic corrugated sheeting and walls of polished timber and bamboo with another wall painted as a large mural, a stunning simplistic image of sub-tropical flora and fauna depicting leaves and insects all hugely over-sized. It was beautifully portrayed, adding to the rustic feel of the place; my gaze returned to it, often.

Most tables were taken and there was a gentle hum of conversation in the back-ground. We settled ourselves at the table offered by the waiter, dressed in black trousers and white shirt. He smiled and chatted to us in English, explaining the various dishes on the menu. After much discussion and deliberation, we made our choices and whilst we waited for our food to be served, the waiter brought us drinks, and as tired and hungry as we were, we found ourselves opening up a little about our backgrounds and why each of us was there, in Baguio.

Chapter 7

Hotel to Green Valley

Eager for the day to begin, my bag slipped onto my shoulder; quietly I pulled the hotel door behind me and went down to the foyer. I was the first to arrive. One by one they joined me. Andrew then Hannah, Greg then Ellen and after much discussion and deliberation, one or two of them would disappear to collect something they had forgotten, or decided they needed, a jacket, a jumper or maybe a mac. We were unsure of the weather and it was chillier than we had anticipated.

"Good morning. Did you all sleep well? Is everybody ready?" called a voice. Paul was holding the door open for us to walk past him and into the waiting mini bus parked on the road. He jumped in with a smile on his face, and said to the driver "All present and correct. Let's go".

This was it. This really was going to be the day when I would meet him, and I would see with my own eyes the wonder of him. I almost had to pinch myself. I looked around at Greg who was looking out of the window taking in the view. Ellen was staring into her lap. There was an almost tangible quietness as each one of us prepared ourselves and tended to our own inner-beings.

I barely noticed our surrounds as we drove from urban to suburban, a mix of apartments and two or three storied homes with balconies. Pine trees grew aplenty thriving well along-side mango trees in the sub-tropical climate.

And then the tarmacadam surface of the road became potholed and less stable, and where the road began to narrow, the land beside the properties fell away on the left, revealing the horse-shoe shape of the mountain terrain. Down in the valley, homes were rooting themselves into the mountainside and were altogether more shanty and hobbled together. Beyond them, the little landing strip of the airport at which we had landed the previous day. The sun was shining, but the distant ridge of the mountain range was shrouded in mist.

On the right-hand side properties were built high up into the hillside. The styles and structures were a strange combination, often of simple breeze block, balconies and flat roofs. Others were reminiscent of Swiss chalets with over-projected roofs to protect the occupants from the weather, or, traditional modern British estate houses of red brick and white window frames. The lavish gardens to these homes were tremendously steep, having high gradient steps to be climbed amongst a plethora of telephone and electricity poles sprouting cable upon cable, causing disturbance to the visual senses.

Somehow, this diverse assortment of dwellings, should never have worked, but in its own way, it did, and carried its own aesthetic beauty. It was intriguing and charming.

Chapter 8

Meeting Roger

The vehicle slowed then came to a halt.

We were outside what seemed to be a café, with a wall painted bubble-gum pink, and bi-fold doors cast open directly onto a concrete paving area.

Without warning, without fanfare, there he was! A tall, good-looking man with straight, shiny, jet-black hair, dark eyes and a broad well-maintained figure, his arms folded. As soon as he saw us, his face broke into a wide warm smile and he stepped forward and pulled open the door of the minibus. Paul stepped out first and shook the man by the hand. As we each individually stepped down onto the concrete, Paul announced our names in turn as Roger shook us by the hand. He was pleased to meet us, and I was thrilled to meet him.

Paul then turned to us all and said, "This is Roger".

Here he was, the man I had travelled half way round the world to meet, standing right in front of me. The moment had arrived. He did not look extraordinary; he had no halo, nor wings. In fact, he looked perfectly normal. What had I been expecting?

In good English, Roger ushered us inside and invited us to sit at the table and enjoy breakfast.

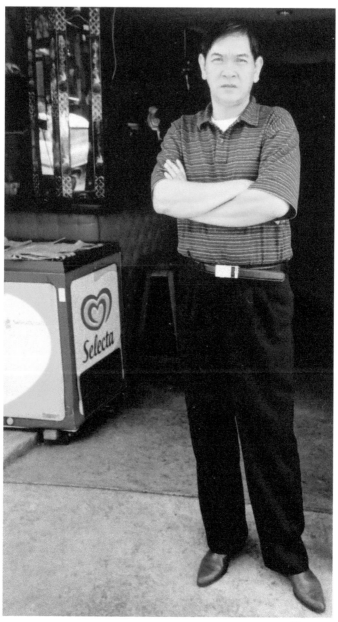

Roger

Chapter 9

The Café

I wasn't aware that I'd had any pre-conceived ideas of the place we were now entering. I actually hadn't really given it too much thought, it hadn't seemed important, but clearly, on some level, I must have had some expectations. I knew we would be eating breakfast here, Paul had said so, and it had always been part of the plan. Yet, could this really be the place I had travelled almost half-way round the world for help? Perhaps this would just be the place we would eat?

As I was absorbing the scene, a short well-bosomed lady with the cheeriest smile and quite glamorous face and dark hair came bustling through a back doorway. She scanned us all and then looked at Paul, and grabbed hold of him, still smiling and gave him the warmest of hugs. Paul hugged her and smiled back. He continued to look at her, and then turned to us and said "Let me introduce Maria, and Maria this is Greg and Ellen, Andrew and Hannah, and Theresa" he continued as one by one we shook hands. "This is Maria's café and she will be cooking for us all whilst you are here in Green Valley". Maria stood erect and beamed, proud of her café. "Hello and welcome, please sit down and I will begin to bring you your breakfast". Her English was impressive.

Two long tables, overlaid with blue and white gingham tablecloths, had been set, one for us and the other for any customers who would call in off the street for a meal, coffee or something stronger. We sat on aqua green plastic garden chairs and drank water that Hannah poured from the freshly filled jugs Maria was placing on the table. Roger joined us.

Whilst the others were making polite conversation (we were still getting to know each other better), I found myself zoning out, fascinated by my surroundings. None of it really computed for me and I was trying to make sense of it all. The wall, the ceiling and the shelves, all painted dark brown, created a dark and dull heavy space. Relief from this darkness came from the hotchpotch of eclectic artefacts, a real mishmash of ornaments and decorations, fruit, fabrics, glass cabinets, flags and plaster-of-paris fish, religious icons, books and masks. At the far end of the room, was a small glass window which looked out onto the white blockwork of an extension being built to the rear of the café. The entirety of that wall was festooned with draped white net curtains, below which was a kind of cupboard covered in an oatmeal cloth topped with red fabric, and served as a display area or alter for scattered fruit and flowers, resembling harvest festival.

I watched as Maria brought to the table, home-mixed muesli, plates of mangos, bananas, toast, juice and coffee. She kept disappearing behind a tall counter bringing everything to the table on trays. The front of the bar was covered in red quilted plastic, edged with black vinyl and the counter was red glass. Had the bar been less cluttered, and not quite so high, she could have used that as a half-way house for all that she was carrying back and forth.

For a moment I had disappeared into my own observational world but was soon pulled back into the conversation around the table, as juice and coffee was being poured and muesli and plates of fruit were passed around.

Maria and Roger sat with us at the table, Maria telling us that they were both Catholic, they had three children and had lived in

Green Valley for many years together. Her generous face lit as she told how she loved preparing and cooking for the customers in the café, and mixing with so many visitors from around the world but, she had a problem with her oven which was now old and not working so well. It needed attention but that would have to wait. She would make do. Roger was making light conversation, telling us about the few local facilities and the neighbourhood. The chatter was lively and the energy in the room was tangible. I was full of anticipation and excitement for what would soon happen, but when, how soon?

Each one of us was conscious of waiting for 'the' something to happen. We all knew what, but nobody was mentioning it, except quietly whispering to each other but pretending not to do so. And so we sat watching jeepneys pulling up on the road outside, teeming with passengers both inside, and on top of the roof, clinging to the handrails to stay aboard. They would climb down onto the dusty road clutching plastic carrier bags, and then drift into the few nearby shops hidden from view by a mountain of red plastic Coca-Cola crates, to buy food.

A few customers came in to the café and went up to the bar, and Maria left the table quickly to serve them with cigarettes, or maybe an ice-cream from the cabinet outside on the road. Roger put some music on the sound system and we continued to wait.

Paul had a responsibility to the group, and must have sensed that something needed to change. I heard him ask Roger,"Will you being seeing us today, is there something you are waiting for?"

"Spirit, it will happen, I am waiting to be nudged" he said, "but meanwhile I can do nothing more than wait". A few minutes later he was seen slowly pacing out in the morning sunshine, back and forth. The flow of conversation picked up again, and slowly we each began to reveal our stories and our reason for being there. Our backgrounds were very different but our incentive for being there were equal and it was at that point I felt that we began to come together, to bond, as a group. It felt good, it felt exciting and it also felt very natural and organic.

All of a sudden, and without warning, Roger came in quickly from the sunshine, called to Ellen and Greg to follow him and disappeared from view with the pair of them in tow. The remaining four of us looked at each other and I asked Paul if they would be going first and he said yes, that was the way they wanted it, privately. I walked out to the street finding something to occupy myself when Paul came to me and said that Roger wanted me to join them.

"Why? I asked, "They want to be alone you said".

"He says your energy would help, he wants you in there".

I looked at Hannah, then Andrew, and back again to Paul. A mix of emotions ran through me.

"My *energy*" I asked. "What do you mean?"

"I don't know. He just asked me to ask you to go in as he needed your energy in the room. It would be helpful".

Puzzled and intrigued, I took a deep breath, turned and headed in the direction in which they had disappeared, and was surprised to find I had walked directly into another room. I vaguely recall the impression of walls painted in differing colours, the dark brown floor, and books piled onto shelving, and photographs pinned to a wall. For in the centre of the room, Greg was lying on a healing table which was covered with a purple bath towel and he was lying naked from the waist down, apart from his socks.

Feeling awkward and a little embarrassed, I looked directly at Roger and said "Ummmm, you wanted me here?"

"Yes," Roger said, looking me straight in the eye. "It is important that you know that I am not a cowboy as is sometimes implied about people like me, and I want you to experience this for yourself, and to know; it is important that you 'know'."

I looked at him, and then at Greg lying on the table looking up at me, and then to Ellen. Was she okay with this, I questioned myself, but the decision seemed not to be in her hands. This man was in control.

This man, Roger, whom we had come so far to meet, had a specialism to which few have access. Maybe specialism is not technically the correct word to use, gift would definitely be better, but a gift to which he was only able to gain access when in this particular part of the Philippines. Roger was a psychic bare-hand surgeon. He psychically physically healed people. He healed them with surgery, proper operations. He operated without using knives, scalpels, anaesthesia, without instruments, without pain, with very little recovery time, and truly amazingly, no scarring.

At no point, from the moment I had read the article a couple of years back, had it occurred to me that he was a cowboy. Why would people think that? Why would people be so fearful? Why could they not be open to a world of possibilities? Why could they not just accept? Why do they always want evidence? Whatever happened to trust and inner knowing? I had every confidence that Roger would perform operations on me with no drugs, no pain, no respite time and leaving no scarring whatsoever. I had absolutely no doubt. To me, this seemed as though it was the most natural way of healing, and I had total trust in the process, so much in fact, that I don't think I was capable, at that time, of totally appreciating the awesomeness of him and his gift.

Roger continued "and the first procedure I carry out on men, no matter what else they have come here for, is to clean the prostate. This has to be healthy before I can proceed with anything else and it will benefit the rest of the body," he said, still looking at me.

"Let's start" said Roger, and his hands scanned and hovered lower down Greg's body and within a blink of an eye, Roger had his finger inside Greg's scrotum and was moving his finger around deep within. I watched Greg's face to see if there was any reaction. I wasn't expecting any and there wasn't any. Roger looked at me and said "Here, put your finger in here with me, I want you to feel the difference between an unclean prostate and a clean prostate." Greg was watching me, and when I glanced at Ellen, she had her camera already videoing the procedure.

I looked at Roger, and then at Greg to see if he had any objection, and then at Ellen, this was her husband, after all. They all seemed to be waiting for me to just go ahead. I could never have been a conventional nurse, dealing with all the blood and gore, and I had never really liked touching other peoples' bodies much, but this couldn't have felt more different, more natural. It felt like an absolute honour to be part of this, a very spiritual experience. I felt special. I could never have imagined having such an opportunity.

Roger kept his finger in place, and I slid my middle finger alongside his into the opening he had made into Greg's scrotum. "Now, I want you to move your finger all around the inside, and to push much further back, to the prostate, and to remember how it feels" he said. I did. The skin was thin with fine raised veins and a thin coating of something slightly moist. I had no reference point. "Right", said Roger, "I am going to put some tissue in here for 24 hours to absorb anything that should not be there, and tomorrow I will remove it and you will see what has been removed. And then, I want you to go in again and feel the difference, and you will know that it is clean".

I withdrew my finger and from a box on the shelf, I passed him a couple of paper tissues which he screwed up into a ball and inserted into the opening, and with his left hand, covered his right index finger as he pulled it out of the opening. With a damp cloth, he wiped the blood from the skin. There was no mark, nothing to show what had just happened. This whole process took no more than 2 or 3 minutes. Ellen put her video camera down, happy that she had some footage.

Although there was no external mark, Roger said it was important to honour the surgery and also to give the body time to heal on the inside where the changes were happening. He put his hand onto Greg for a few moments and allowed energy to flow through his own body and through to Greg and then asked that if any of us were healers to do some energy work on him for 15 minutes. Roger placed a blanket across his patient to help him feel cosy and comfortable whilst he was lying there, recuperating. Ellen was a Reiki Master, well used to healing others, and so she sat on a chair behind Greg's head and placed her hands on the sides of his face to maintain the energy flow. Paul came into the room and held Greg's feet and as he also was a Reiki Master and was able to help the flow of energy.

"Greg, with that tissue in you, how does it feel" I asked, unable to imagine what that must be like.

"Uncomfortable right now", said Greg, but as Roger had explained, the soggier the tissue gets, the softer it would become and the more comfortable he would feel.

That was my first and highly memorable experience for me of psychic bare-hand surgery; such an experience. There would be much more to follow.

"Why did you learn Reiki?" I asked both Ellen.

Ellen explained that she had been on a spiritual path over a period of many years. She became actively interested in alternative therapies and modalities but her interest really piqued when she had taken a Reiki course and become a Reiki Master. This gave her the ability to bring relief to many people, including Greg. Greg had held a high position in a company in the scientific field but in recent times had need of some surgery. Through Paul, Greg learnt about Roger, and this seemed the most obvious and logical way to go and even though psychic surgery was so far removed from his own business.

I stood with Ellen and Greg for a few minutes, absorbing the scene and processing what had just happened. It seemed surreal, yet very *real*.

Chapter 11

My First Operation

Back in the café, Roger was drinking water, and the others were drinking fruit juice left over from breakfast. Looking at me curiously, they asked "what happened in there?", and I simply said "I have just felt inside Greg's scrotum, his prostate needed cleaning". They looked at me astonished. "Roger inserted some tissue to absorb any infection that may have been there and tomorrow he will remove it."

Roger stood up and went back into the surgery to check on Greg and to sense whether his internal healing time was completed. After a few minutes, it seemed it had, for he then called us all into the room together, just as Greg was getting himself off the table, lowering himself to the floor and pulling his trousers back on.

"Right, let's get started again. Next", said Roger as he pointed to me.

"You mean for surgery?" I said.

"Yes, quickly, get up here, I have to be quick".

Now, the reason I was up in there in the mountains was because conventional medicine suggested I have major surgery to have an ovarian cyst removed. It had been with me for a number of years and had remained dormant, but would it always? A separate issue was a fibroid which had also grown over the years, maybe since the birth of my children and had now become the size of a fist with extending appendages. The options were to leave things as they were and hope, or to have them removed with the use of anaesthetics and major conventional surgery, or my new option of surgery in the energy vortex here in The Philippines.

Roger was waiting. I leapt up onto the table, fully clothed and Roger pushed my trousers down sufficiently to uncover my stomach, and I removed my top and was then lying on the bed, looking up at all the faces staring down at me. Ellen was standing on a chair she had pulled closer, higher than the rest with her video camera pointing down at me.

Theresa prepared for the operation

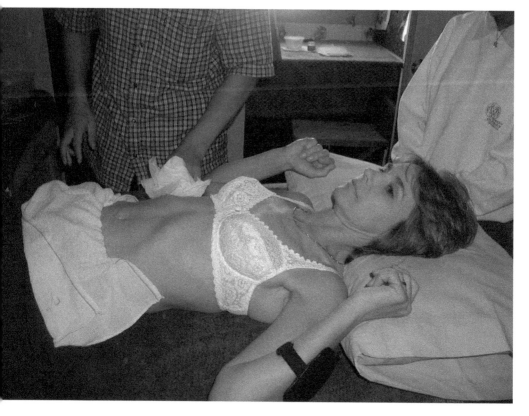

Roger skimmed my body with his hands, sensing the area that needed his intervention and I felt him touch my stomach and looked down and asked what was happening. Andrew said "He's in".

"What, actually in?" I was astonished and amazed. I had not felt anything.

"Yes, look" he said.

I looked down just as Roger was placing on my naval, a thick and bloody piece of fleshy tissue, and the size of a flattened tinned tomato and with tendril like roots attached to one side. He was going back in and tugged out another much smaller piece which he placed next to the first. And then, with his left hand, he covered his right hand and withdrew his finger, and wiped my stomach with a damp cloth. There was no mark, no scar, and no evidence at all of what had just happened. Roger picked up the main piece of flesh, very bloodied, examined it and then showed it to me and all of us. Hannah had been snapping away with her camera, and now both she and Ellen with her video camera, asked Roger for a close-up shot. He happily obliged and began talking to camera about the condition of the flesh. Satisfied that this was healthy tissue, he turned, aimed and threw it in the bin a few feet away. This had been part of the fibroid I had been living with for years.

I was totally conscious, fully awake and able to move every part of my body. I was aware of everything going on around me, participating in conversation and yet I had not felt Roger opening my stomach, inserting his fingers deeply enough to grasp and pull out parts of my body.

"That is not the whole fibroid, Roger, is it?" I asked him. He explained that it would not be possible for him to remove the whole thing in one go, for two reasons, the first being that spirit would not allow him to create an opening large enough to remove the whole thing in one go, and secondly, it would be dangerous because my body would have difficulty recovering from such an extreme removal. It was going to take quite a number of operations, over quite a number of days, before the whole of it was removed.

Suddenly, Roger had penetrated with his finger, the other side of my stomach. Paul was gently holding my wrist. I looked down to watch what was happening, and although I could see a thumb and three fingers, the fourth, index finger had disappeared within me. He then inserted the index finger of his left hand and pulled out another fleshy piece and laid it on me. Sensing there was no more he should remove at that time, he covered his right hand and withdrew his fingers, wiped me with a damp cloth, leaving no mark whatsoever. Again, he picked up the fleshy matter and examined it as Ellen and Hannah were getting clear shots of my inners.

"This", said Roger, "is part of your ovarian cyst and it looks healthy but again it will take several operations to remove it completely. It's okay, we have time" and turned and threw it in the bin.

Even though, in theory, I had known what to expect, the experience of it was more difficult to comprehend. This felt like the most natural, the most normal thing in the world, but at the same time, it was mind-blowing, difficult to absorb. I held his hand in total gratitude, my eyes stinging with tears. "Roger, thank you so much, thank you". The words seemed totally inadequate.

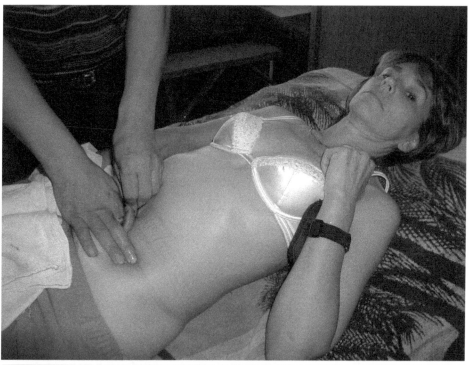

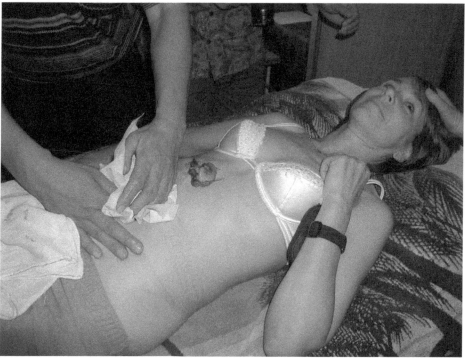

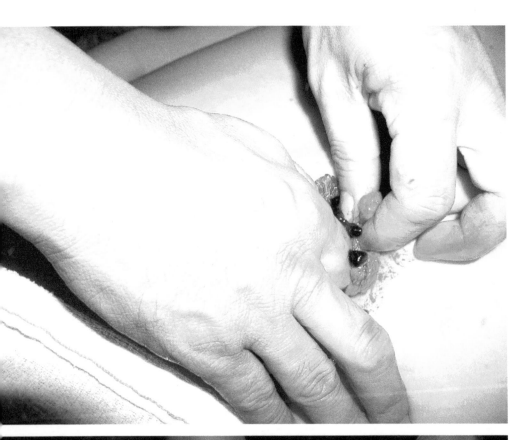

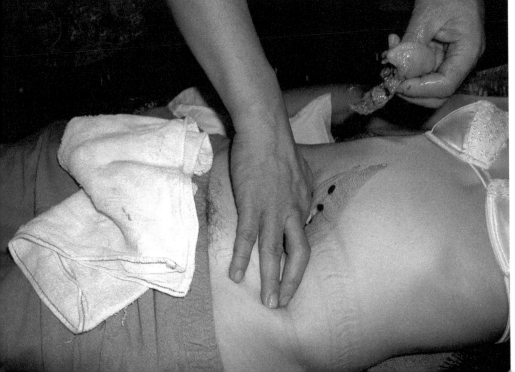

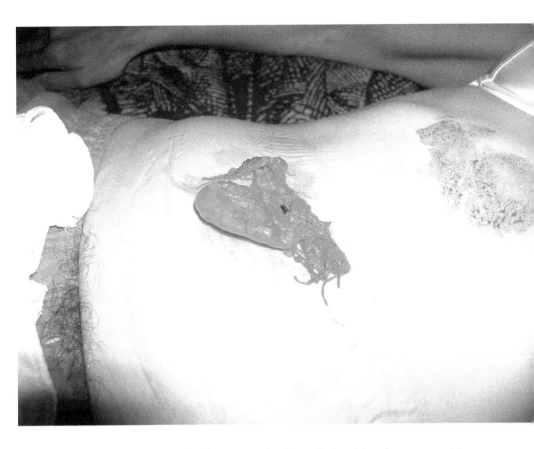

He wiped my stomach clean, and placed the blanket over. He searched into my eyes for a second, held his hands over me and then asked for any of the others who could do healing to do so for me. Ellen stood beside me with her hands on my body, Patrick held my feet and together were sending me energy. Andrew pulled up a chair. He sat close to my head and started to hum. His voice was deep, and I felt the vibration reverberating from him. I lay there facing the ceiling, my eyes closed, totally accepting the love and caring being given to me. Andrew had been humming his own healing energy for a few minutes, and gradually the sound changed to a series of single notes, almost a chant, with the vibration changing accordingly. It was a serene and magical moment for all of us.

A quarter of an hour had passed when the room filled again. Roger, followed by Hannah and Greg all filed in. Roger stood and sensed the energy of my body, and released me from the table. Before my feet had touched the ground, he indicated to Hannah that she would be next and tapped the table quickly.

Hannah backed herself up onto the table and adjusted the pillow beneath her head. Before she could say anything, Roger told her to remove her top, he needed to operate. His hands hovered over her collar bone below the centre of her neck, then his fingers touched her skin and instantly his finger had made an opening as he slid it inside. Immediately, he pulled out a cream and red long, round, worm-like shape, about two and a half inches long and held it up for her to see.

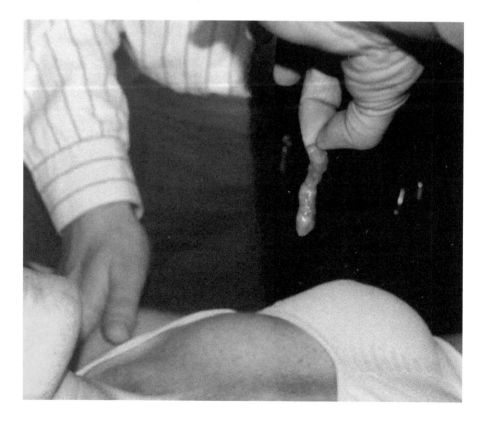

I needed to record the wonders that I was seeing, and was standing on the opposite side of the bed to Roger taking my own photographs. Ellen was positioned on the chair and was filming the whole proceedings on video.

But Hannah was fascinated with what he had just pulled out from her, and gently took it from him. She held it between her fingers, gingerly touching it with a bemused and happy smile on her face.

"What actually is it? She asked. Roger explained that in the past she may have had an accident and been hit in the chest, and this was the matter that had built up causing a blockage. Hannah recalled an incident earlier in her life, so this made perfect sense to her.

"Thank you, Roger, thank you" she said, patting his arm in gratitude, "Thank you".

Roger nodded his acknowledgement and with a white paper tissue took the fleshy matter from her and held it out for us to photograph "It is important that you capture this well" he said before throwing that too into the bin.

"Now", said Roger, "turn onto your side, there is a problem behind your ear". Hannah turned and lay on her left side and Roger began scanning her head, hovering with his hands. He reached up to the table beside him and pulled a cocktail stick from a container and turned to Hannah. We all looked at each other. "Surely not" we silently thought. But yes, he pushed the cocktail stick into and through the skull behind her ear, and somehow pulled out some bloody red matter, reinserted it and pulled out more. Sliding a finger into flesh was one thing, but a piece of wood through the skull quite another.

Roger finished and covered the opening with his left hand,

again, leaving no trace of this surgery, and left the room for a moment. He returned with a spring onion in his hand. He had cut away the rooted end leaving a six inch long stem and he placed it in Hannah's ear. She looked at him, startled and began giggling. "Leave it there for 15 minutes. It will help to cleanse deep into the ear and skull" he said. "You need to do this, and yes, I know it's funny". By now we were all giggling. There she was lying on a table in her trousers and bra with a spring onion sticking from her ear!

With great intensity working with spirit, Hannah had only been up on the table for about five or six minutes. Then as was becoming the normal part of the procedure she was covered with a blanket whilst her husband gave vibrational voice healing at her head and Paul delivered his own healing at her feet.

Chapter 12

Taking Responsibility

Meanwhile, Roger had taken himself into the café, and we could hear him talking in Filipino, to another man and they seemed comfortable in each other's company with much laughter and banter between them. And then it stopped. Roger appeared alongside the table to check on Hannah and said "Yes, you're okay, you can get up now and I think we should break for coffee. I need a break before spirit will let me continue".

That seemed like a good plan to me. I needed a little time to integrate what had happened that morning, to absorb the energy to try to comprehend the awesomeness of it all. How does one comprehend that a man can make an opening in somebody's flesh simply with his finger, with no pressure, no drugs, no tools except maybe a toothpick and some tissues and pull out pieces of flesh, with no pain? We had seen and experienced something miraculous and organic – we had seen the truth and the reality with our own eyes. I just accepted it for the natural healing that it was, plain and simple.

The friend was nowhere to be seen. Roger was sitting at a table avidly reading the front page of the local paper, keeping abreast of what had been happening in his neighbourhood. Maria was busying herself with the coffee, and cutlery and crockery that seemed to be needed. She placed a large jug of filtered coffee on the table, enough for us all, and a vacuum flask of extra coffee, just in case. Milk came in the form of powdered milk, from a tin.

Ellen poured coffee for everybody and passed round the tin of milk, should anybody wish to use it. I looked at Paul and asked him why there wasn't any real milk adding that coffee was not the same without real milk.

"Well", Paul said, "Now that you are here and having these treatments, and also when you get back home, I would suggest you be on a macrobiotic diet".

"Macrobiotic? What do you mean, what would that mean for me? Why?" I was full of questions.

"Well, part of the reason you are here is because of your diet and the other reason is probably emotional blockages. You have created your fibroid. You don't want your condition to return, so you are going to have to make a change to your diet. Your body needs to be alkaline." Roger continued "It is important to realise the problems the wrong foods can cause to your body, the blockages they can create and the tumours that are formed. You have already seen for yourself what I mean by that".

"So no meat, no dairy, no cheese, no fish" said Paul, and continued "I used to love sushi, I ate lots of it, but then I discovered cancerous tumours on my liver caused partly by the sushi. I no longer eat fish of any kind. I am totally macrobiotic and just about cured, but I will continue with the diet, to be sure".

Gosh, the diet didn't sound very appealing, quite harsh in fact but Maria had produced some delicious food for breakfast so perhaps it would be easier with some practice but I knew I would have the urge for some chocolate.

"Paul... I know that at some point I will really want some choco..." and before I could finish the sentence, Paul interrupted, with an amused but firm "No!"

We sat quietly for a few minutes, drinking our coffee, listening to the noise of the traffic outside, and some music coming quietly from somewhere behind the counter. A man went up to the bar and asked Maria for a packet of cigarettes and a take away coffee, and a young mother bought her toddling daughter an ice cream, and they sat together on the plastic chairs outside on the pavement.

Three of us had experienced surgery now, but also had Paul on his previous visits to this clinic, and he would be having more. Hopefully, this morning, Ellen and Andrew at least would receive some treatment.

Chapter 13

Preconceived Notions

Roger leapt up from his chair, and walked into the lavatory, barely closing the door behind him whilst he spent a penny. I was slightly taken aback, and even more so when I noticed that when he had finished he had not washed his hands, and walked straight into the surgery. I was quite fastidious about personal hygiene and particularly hand washing. This didn't quite add up considering our circumstances and I was trying to reconcile my own standards with his, only to be distracted by a grey mouse scurrying along the skirting board, pass the lavatory and into the surgery!

"Ah! Roger", I called out walking in towards him. "A mouse has just run into the surgery".

Roger looked at me as I looked at him, expecting some kind of reaction. He vaguely glanced at the floor, shrugged his shoulders and straightened the blanket on the bed. The others hearing what I had said, followed me quickly into the room, picking up and moving things, hoping to find the mouse. Roger was completely unperturbed.

"Let's get started Andrew" he said and pointed to the table.

At that point, I was completely accepting of whatever happened up there in the mountains, none of it equated with the reality I once knew. Spirit was everything, and everything was possible. What was the deal with our perceived idea of hygiene and a little mouse running around the room? Here, it was irrelevant.

Andrew was about to lie down on the table when Roger asked him to remove his trousers and his underpants. First, he was going to clean his prostate! We all looked at Andrew, and then to Hannah. Andrew removed the said clothing and removed his tee shirt also, and was back on the bed completely naked. He did not seem uncomfortable with us all standing around, looking at him. Ellen was standing with her video camera aimed towards him and started to film and I picked up my own camera. It felt important to record as much of these procedures as possible, for reminders in the future.

Roger began scanning Andrew's groin and swiftly entered his scrotum and created an opening with his right index finger. His finger buried deep within as he felt and gauged the condition. Hannah's intention to photograph her husband disappeared as she was examining closely the work Roger was doing. She handed him a white paper tissue from a box on the table. He loosely screwed it up, placed another finger into the scrotum to widen the hole, then placed the tissue inside, and as he was about to withdrew his finger he covered it with his left hand. With a damp cloth Roger wiped away the blood, and told Andrew that the following day he would remove the tissue, but it may be a little uncomfortable overnight. Hannah was simply standing there, riveted.

Hannah and Andrew had problems with conception. With her advancing years in terms of pregnancy, she was desperate to have a baby, mothering instinct had been coursing through her being for a few years, and as each month passed, each month brought disappointment. She and Andrew were grasping a final, possible chance, here in Baguio with Roger. And now she was looking at her husband's manhood, packed full of tissue paper!

Roger was looking at her, and was reading her mind. "We are dealing with a basic issue here", he said to her, "until the prostate is clean and healthy, then there is no point in continuing elsewhere. Patience, we will try and get you pregnant, if that is what is meant to be", he continued.

Hannah surrendered her feelings to his higher wisdom, and remembered to breath. She took a slow, deep, long breath as she assimilated this experience with her husband, and her mood changed as she sensed that her world was beginning to open up to new possibilities. She covered Andrew, pulled up a chair beside him, and we left them together whilst his body healed.

"Ellen, you're next. Please be up on the table", Roger was saying as he pulled the blanket straight. The same blanket we had all lain on for our operations. Ellen pulled herself up onto the table and Roger asked her to lower her trousers a little, but she removed them altogether and lay there in her underwear. Greg, in dark navy blue trousers, and blue short sleeved checked shirt, climbed up onto the chair with the video camera. The frame of his brown rimmed glasses was proving to be a little problematic, but he eventually found a way that worked for him and with which he was comfortable. Whatever was about to happen, he wanted to record it, so that in the future he would realise this had not all been just a dream.

We, again, all gathered around the table. Roger was soon scanning Ellen's body, hovered over her stomach, and within a blink of an eye, had two fingers digging deep into her flesh. He was feeling around her deep intestines, and pulling and pulling, until finally he held up something that resembled a caterpillar, complete with head, deep red in colour, covered in blood. Ellen looked aghast.

"What is THAT?" she asked.

"That", replied Roger with his finger still in the opening "was a blockage in your large intestine, trapped on a bend, and little has been able to pass through". He was back inside again, prodding and pulling, and he brought out another piece, different in shape, softer, but could easily have filled the palm of her hand.

"And this is a growth which shouldn't be there" he said as he was scrutinising the bloody matter. He covered his finger and withdrew it to close the opening, and wiped her body clean of all blood. He then pulled a knife from his pocket, cut the growth in half down the centre, and opened it up to reveal a length of pale grey interior.

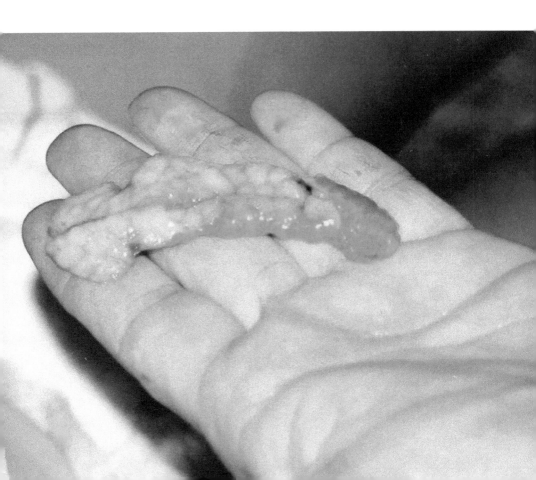

"Hmmm, you were lucky there" he said "this is cancer. This is all I will do for today, but I will investigate again next time". So, this is what cancer looked like, and Roger had just removed it from her body.

"Oh! My goodness, thank you Roger, thank you so much, but what caused it?" she asked looking up to him.

"Apart from maybe some emotional issues, this was caused by diet, probably too much cheese and dairy which takes the longest time to break down, and meat isn't any better" he replied. "You can choose to do differently now. Meanwhile, just lay there quietly".

Andrew again pulled his chair up close to Ellen and began to softly hum in her ear. Greg stood with his hands on her stomach, reflecting on what he had just witnessed. I sat quietly, listening to the deep, caressing tones of Andrew's voice. He hummed each velvety rich note with total control, and it drove deep into my core. The hairs on the back of my neck stood on end. I shivered and was captivated by the moment.

Ellen, Andrew and Greg had left the room. "Just coming", I called after them as they left the room. I sat alone in the "surgery". I needed to be alone to embrace all that happened that morning. This all seemed so natural to me, so totally, amazingly natural.

I looked around the room, at the "surgery". It was a small room, about the size of an average dining room, with a small window allowing in just sufficient light. The only thing that resembled a "surgery" to me was the white ceiling, which would have benefitted from a coat of paint. The walls were roughly plastered and painted a bright deep golden yellow, now, sadly peeling away from the walls, and the supporting joists around the room painted turquoise. The door opening from the cafe was grass green surrounded with black architrave and the beams

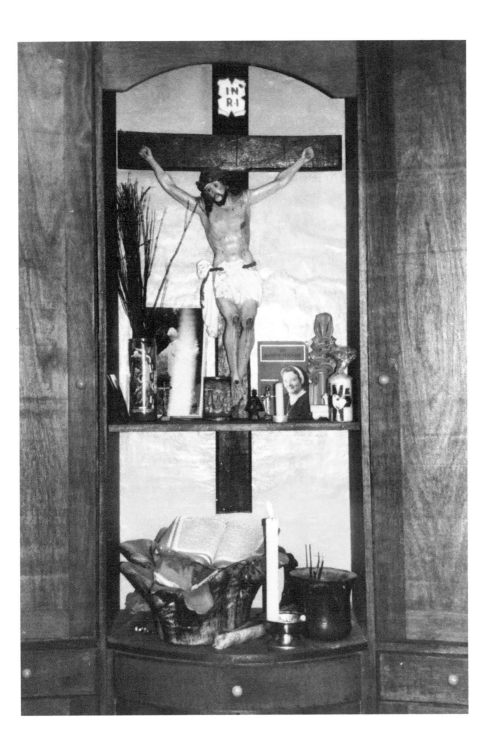

supporting the ceiling were painted black or turquoise. Hanging from these golden walls, hung a circular tray with religious icons, and various simple paintings placed in random fashion.

Beside the door stood two tall teak cupboards connected by a shorter cupboard and a shelf fitted between them on which was an image of Jesus on a dark wooden cross. This little area was dedicated as a temple, and a candle flickered. An assortment of sentimental items were placed, muddled, on this temple, including a photograph of a nun, and one of my own daughter which I had given to Roger earlier. It felt important that she be part of this experience and she constantly let me know that she was.

A long pin board was covered with photographs of the people on whom Roger had performed operations. Dozens and dozens, some of them with notes and letters attached. It was fascinating seeing all the faces looking at me, looking into the room they had known so well, and as I was getting to know it too. This was a true board of gratitude.

On the far side of the room a table upon which Roger kept his surgical instruments; a box of white tissues (we had all been asked to bring a contribution), cotton buds and cocktail sticks. No anaesthesia, no instruments, no oxygen masks, in fact, nothing clinical whatsoever.

Alongside the window, a door opened into a tiny room with a basin, a bucket and an open-topped bin, into which Roger threw our flesh. "Was the mouse in there?" I thought, remembering it had not yet been found.

"Are you coming, Theresa?" called Paul, "we can stay for lunch and go for a walk in the park later if you would like to do that". I was jolted from my own inner world and my attention brought back to theirs, and joined them.

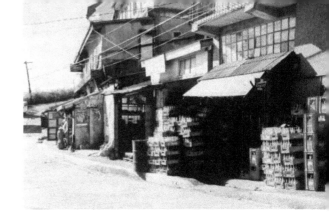

Chapter 14

Café Road

The afternoon was free time, nothing had been planned, and we had not expected that we would stay for lunch. However, Maria had wanted us to stay. She loved a crowd, and was very sociable, but she needed a little time to prepare lunch for us all, and left us to entertain ourselves.

I needed some fresh air and wandered out into the sunshine. It still was not particularly warm and I was grateful for the jumper I had brought with me.

Along the road there was a patchwork of facades to the front elevations of the buildings. Those nearby were commercial with a myriad of cables attached to telegraph poles whilst further along, metal doors and vivid blue plastic awnings projected out onto the road. Flimsy galvanised metal gates pretended to bravely secure some premises, whilst more corrugated plastic sheeting was curved round timber structures to create privacy. Propane gas cylinders, and air conditioning units, scaffolding and stacks of Coca-Cola crates were stacked roof high. It begged the question as to how such a small community could drink such a huge quantity of the coke.

Open-backed trucks rattled along the road on their way to deliver construction materials to building sites. Other delivery vehicles dropped off vegetables at the greengrocers, or tins and packets to the general store to keep the little shop well stocked. Cheerful and brightly coloured jeepneys were fun to watch, as the number of people crammed both inside and on top was amazing. There seemed to be a constant flow of passengers to drop off or collect.

My thoughts were disrupted and my attention was driven towards an incident happening outside a store selling household goods, and adjoining what looked to be a cave. Bent forward and running along the pavement were half a dozen young men. They were dragging a pig and had tied its snout up with string, using it as a lead and were yelling at it and tapping its trotters with a hockey stick to encourage it to move along. The pig was grunting and snorting, refusing to move any further, but the men yelled louder, pulled harder and tapped faster until eventually the pig went with them and climbed up a steep flight of concrete steps. At the top, more people were waiting for the pig to arrive to escort it into a butchery for slaughter. It was an upsetting scene, and I felt disturbed. For the pig this was such an inhumane way for it to end its short life, frightened and without choice and all because customers wanted the freshest of meat, all be it now with the energy of fear embedded within its carcass.

I was heading back to the café, and almost there, when further down the road I could see the school bus unloading. I was surprised the children were home so early, perhaps today was just a half-day? Soon, little groups of them swarmed pass me. They were a delight.

The young girls with glossy black hair were sweetly dressed in their loosely pleated uniform jade green skirts, held up by wide jade green fabric braces over white blouses, and topped with deep rose coloured cardigans. Some wore black winter shoes with white socks, whilst some wore simple flip-flops. Walking hand in hand, the girls enjoyed each other's company and laughed and chatted with the ease that comes with great friendship. As they passed they smiled at me, looked at each, giggled together and skipped off.

The boys seemed not to wear a uniform but jeans, tee shirts and anoraks, and wearing trainers seemed to be the order of the day. These boys rough and tumbled their way, with little teasing fights breaking out and then bursting into laughter. They could see me watching them and smiled at me but seemed less confident than the girls. Within a few minutes of them jumping down from the bus, filling the street with their chatter and laughter and bringing life and energy to the mountainside, they vanished as quickly as they had appeared.

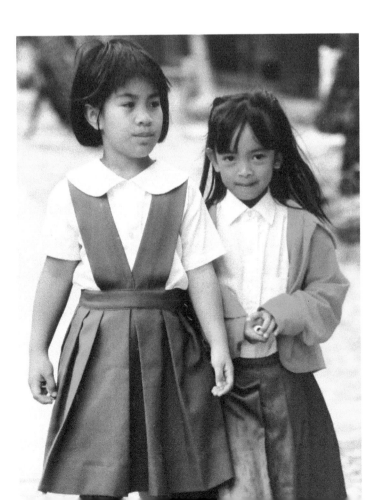

Chapter 15

Free Time

Through into the café, I could see the men sitting at the table, staring intently at one of the video cameras, watching some of the footage from earlier. They hardly noticed me, but I stood over and joined them. The images were very clear, and they had managed to get sharp shots of Roger's fingers deep in the flesh and all the matter he was pulling out. There were so many scenes and it was good to revisit that which we had just experienced for ourselves, now being able to switch between scenes and fully study what had taken place.

Ellen and Hannah appeared, nattering together as Maria set the table. Roger carried a large bowl of rice, and Maria brought a dish of stir-fried vegetables. She sat with us, chatting and laughing, explaining enthusiastically about how she had cooked the stir-fry, what ingredients she had used plus a secret ingredient which she was not going to share! There was a warmth and sparkle in her eyes as she was telling us her stories. We all listened intently before turning our attention to the meal Maria had prepared. I hadn't known how hungry I was until I saw the food, all good and healthy, and we all delved in.

Fully satiated and sitting with our coffee Roger was asked how he came to be serving humanity with this psychic bare-hand surgery.

"Well" he said, "when I was still of school age, I was with a friend who began to choke and was struggling to breath and would die, I knew he would die. There was panic. The next thing I found myself reaching through his neck and pulled out the obstruction and there was no pain for him and no evidence of what had happened. He was shocked and grateful, as you can imagine, but for me it was extremely scary and I was afraid and frightened about what I had just done, I didn't understand the experience, and I ran off into the woods and stayed there for many days before returning home to my family. I did not understand my gift then. Afterwards, I went on to study the theory of medicine in order that I had some understanding of human anatomy and the metaphysical body and that was when I began to practice".

With lunch over Roger drove us back to our hotel to freshen up. Fortunately, his vehicle was large enough to accommodate us all. He dropped us off and we agreed to rest a while. I had underestimated how energy sapping the morning had been. The simple participation of laying down and receiving operations, the post-operative healing, watching others and their operations and recording each of the events, brought to the fore deep emotions which needed to be processed. A rest was very welcome.

The plan was to go to the park, to walk, to commune with nature. I felt that for the past two days all I had seemed to do was sit, and my legs were definitely in need of some exercise. But Greg and Ellen said they would like to go shopping and take some time out. There was something special they would like to do and called a taxi to take them into the City. We took a taxi of our own to one of the small local parks and watched the children on the boating lake shouting and laughing at each other. Pine trees shaded areas of the park, and benches had been placed for people to be able to sit quietly and enjoy the exotic gardens.

Eventually we had dawdled back to the gate and Paul's phone rang. Greg and Ellen had finished their shopping and wanted to meet for an early evening meal. They would come and find us; they were on their way.

Very soon, a cab pulled alongside and the pair of them stepped out. Paul knew exactly the right place to take us to eat, just along the road. The restaurant was typical Filipino, and with a good range of vegetarian dishes. Paul had eaten there often. We scoured and analysed the menu and would have liked to have been more adventurous, but our new diet would not allow such a thing. A glass of wine, and twenty minutes later, we placed our order, and waited.

"Ellen" I said to her, "what was it you needed in the City, something special? Whatever it was, you seem pretty pleased with yourself. Going to share?" I said, teasingly and laughing.

She looked at Greg for approval, but then couldn't hold back. "Well, actually, we went shopping for an oven".

"An *oven*!" I repeated, had I heard correctly? "An oven! What would you need an oven for here?"

"We don't" she said, "but we thought we would buy one for Maria. "She was explaining the problems she was having with her oven. With the cost of the building work they are having done, buying an oven is way down on their list of priorities. I tried to find out what she would like from a new oven, but she wasn't very forthcoming, so we thought we would just buy one for her, it's not as though we can't afford it".

We all looked at her and then at Greg and we could see they had a real sense of satisfaction to be able to do that for her. It was such a generous idea to actually go and buy it.

"It is going to be delivered tomorrow lunch time, just after we have finished surgery, so, don't tell her, let's just keep it between ourselves, a secret" she said. We all happily agreed and looked forward to its arrival.

Maria and Roger at their café

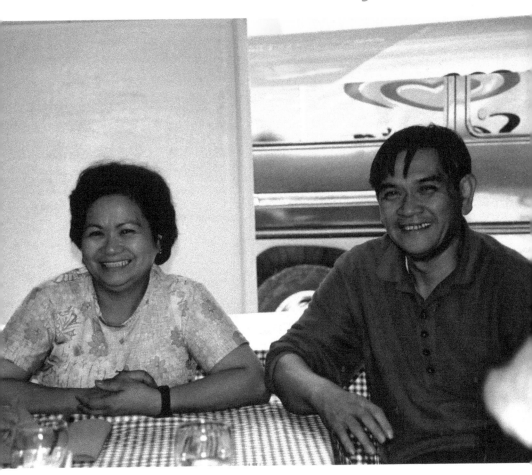

Chapter 16

Men's Department

The following morning, Roger came to the hotel, his mood was light and airy, he gathered us all up and twenty minutes later we piled out of his dark silver 4x4. Maria, dressed in black trousers and a simple purple blouse, beamed at us and hugged us one by one.

The table was set. White tablecloths with poppies printed around the edge and upturned glasses were already laid out for us, together with jugs filled with apple juice so that we could help ourselves.

"Take a seat, sit yourselves down, coffee is on its way. Would anybody like porridge this morning?" she asked.

Up in the mountain, there was still a nip in the air, and porridge had great appeal. Maria served each of us full bowls which we topped with honey and nuts. Fresh fruit was loosely scattered around the table, platefuls of toast appeared followed by jugs of hot coffee and powdered milk.

The next half an hour was spent fully consumed with breakfast, and as we sat with our second round of coffee Roger and Maria between them brought us up to speed with the overnight politics of the neighbourhood, my thoughts were returning to what would soon be happening.

"How are you feeling this morning Greg" I whispered to him, "is it more comfortable?"

"Actually, yes, much better than last evening when I was quite aware of it, but after a good night's sleep, yes, it feels a lot better. Let's hope that's a good sign" Greg responded.

Only twenty-four hours earlier, I had felt inside Greg's scrotum, now full of tissue paper. "What would that look like today?" I thought "and would Roger really want me to feel inside again?" I felt a little nervous now that I knew what to expect, but what was I really nervous about, I wondered, and then realised I was nervous in case I was disappointed and was not asked.

The wait was not long. Roger had been chatting away to the men, with both his arms on the table, leaning forward with his chin almost resting on them. Suddenly he straightened, stood up, pushed the chair back from behind him and pointed to Greg to follow him into the surgery. We all followed.

Roger directed Greg to remove his trousers and underpants and to get up on the table. Ellen was holding the video camera. "Let's get started" said Roger as his hands hovered above Greg's nether regions. Roger was looking intently as he placed both his fore fingers on the scrotum, dug deeply into the flesh and made an opening. He pulled the opening apart with both fingers, inserted his thumb and pulled out the tissue from the day before. Holding up the bloody mess, he pointed out the gunk which had attached itself to the tissue.

Looking at Greg, and also making sure this was being filmed, Roger pointed, "Here, this is toxic, and could have caused a serious infection, and could have led to prostate cancer" he said, and then threw the tissue in the bin.

"Theresa", said Roger, "I'd like you to insert your finger, as you did yesterday, go up towards the back and run the pad of your finger across the flesh, as before, and notice the difference in texture". I did as I was asked, and allowed the pad of my finger to feel its way back and around the wall. Yes, there certainly was a difference; it felt cleaner and drier is the best way I could describe it.

Satisfied that I was aware of the difference, he withdrew his forefinger from Greg, covered it with his left hand and wiped the area clean, leaving no visible mark whatsoever. He continued to his body, and hovered in one place for a second or two.

Ellen had put the video camera down. I picked it up and continued recording.

"Whilst you have your trousers off, turn over". His hands went straight to Greg's coccyx and hovered, moved slightly further down and with his forefinger probed into the rectum deeply, inserted his thumb and after some seconds, was pulling a length of what Roger described as lactose, similar in looks to a fine tapeworm, creamy in colour beneath the blood. Still holding on to one end of it, Roger continued to pull, and pulled some more.

"I have to be really careful here, if this breaks, I am not going to be able to reach the piece that it has broken from, I have to keep pulling very smoothly. He continued pulling, and pulling, until eventually there was a length, more than a meter long.

"This", he said with a distasteful look on his face," is a result of eating meat and cheese, particularly red meat, pork, beef, lamb. It is too rich and too difficult for the body to absorb and break down the matter. Our bodies are not designed to cope with such food, and this is the result. And actually, not too many western doctors would even recognise what was pulled out. They would not have seen it in a complete length because they do not pull it out like this". He tried flicking it from his arm shaking it violently to get it off and let it fall into the bin. Immediately he wretched forward and threw up!

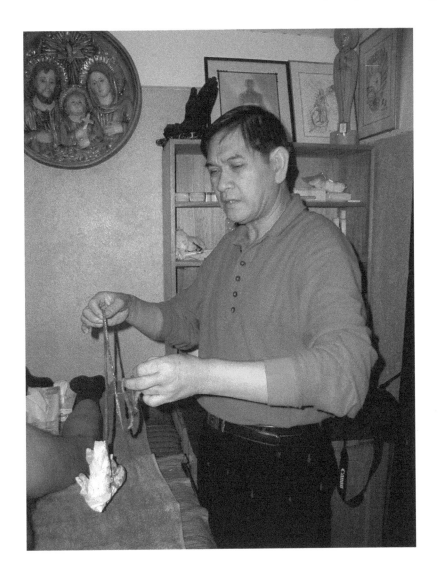

"That was disgusting!" he exclaimed. "Turn on to your side, there is something going on with your thigh, let me see" he continued. Again, his hands hovered over the top of Greg's thigh, and he was in. He had penetrated the flesh with his right forefinger and then his thumb, withdrew a clot and flicked it aside with his fingernail.

Greg pulled himself up, supporting himself with one arm, "That was where I was involved in a motor-bike accident years ago in my twenties, and it has always been a problem. There is often some pain there, but I have just learnt to live with it" Greg stated.

"Now that we have it out, it shouldn't cause you a problem anymore" Roger replied. "You need to rest a while. Ellen, give him some healing please. You too Andrew, he's going to need it. He has had a lot done this morning." Roger covered him with what looked like an old big patterned curtain, and left the room.

Soon after, Roger returned, checked Greg to check that he had internally healed, and released him from the table.

"Andrew, you're next" I heard Roger say, and picked up the camera, ready to take some still shots. Ellen was holding her video camera. Andrew simply removed his clothes and climbed onto the table. Hannah automatically held his hand. Roger went straight to the groin area, hovered his hands, and went straight into the scrotum with two fingers and thumb and pulled out the tissue he had placed there the day before. He studied it and said "There, that doesn't look too bad, but it is better to know it is healthy before we do any other work. He put his finger further in and felt around and checked the prostate. All was well, he was happy, and Roger removed his finger, again, leaving no trace.

"Well, that is good news" said Hannah, "at least we know that is one problem we can eliminate. What else is next?

"Let's see what spirit finds", he said, scanning Andrew's body. Almost instantly, his finger was pushing through the flesh above the pubic bone and he was grappling inside trying to get a grip of something, and with the nail of his other index finger inside, he levered out a length of nine peanut sized gristly balls connected by tissue measuring about six inches long. He held it up for the camera, and also for Andrew to see. Hannah took it from Roger, not quite believing what she was seeing and needed to hold it and feel it and smell it for herself, to help to more easily understand what she was seeing.

"What is that?" cried Andrew. "Where was it?"

"I am not sure I can give it a name, but it was clogging up your lower intestine, caught on a bend, creating a blockage. It can be caused by two things; the food you have eaten and the emotional blockages which have not been released" he explained. "Your system is going to feel a whole lot better now it has been removed". His finger had been keeping the opening open, but he withdrew it whilst it was covered by his left hand and, without drawing breath, moved across his body and made another opening, and inserted two fingers. He felt around until he located another problem. With both fingers and his thumb, he pulled out more matter. Before Andrew could ask, he said "and this is another blockage in your large intestine", and showed it to camera. It looked like pieces of liver connected by loose tissue. He laid it on his body for inspection. We all looked at it quizzically, not really understanding, before it was discarded to the bin.

"That is enough for this morning Andrew, you need to heal, I will be back in a while". Roger disappeared into the café. Paul and Ellen sat either side of Andrew, quietly sending healing to his body, and taking the opportunity to quietly give thanks and to embrace the energy surrounding them.

Twenty minutes later, with a new sense of urgency, Roger returned, looked at Hannah, and indicated that he wanted her up next. Andrew lowered himself from the table and Hannah replaced him.

Roger returned to Hannah's neck and removed some more matter from her chest.

"Turn over" he said "there is more to do on your back". Hannah turned and he scanned her shoulder and was soon removing more matter. Roger then closed the opening and placed the flesh on tissue to show her what he had removed, before wiping her back clean.

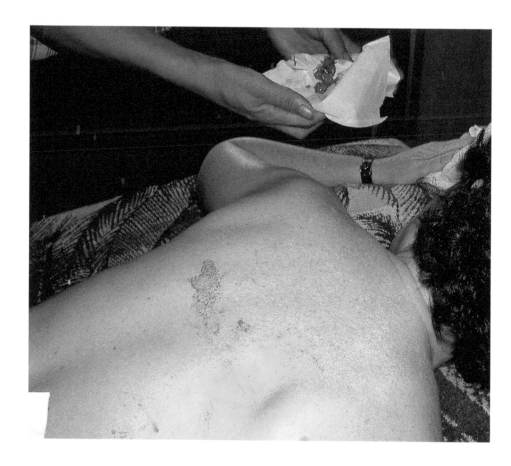

I was up next and had more of my fibroid and ovarian cyst removed and Paul had a routine partial liver tumour removed. It was then lunch time. Roger asked that we stay on for the afternoon, as he wanted to perform more operations, and he was really only touching the tip of the iceberg, and there was plenty more to do.

We stayed for lunch. Maria had been preparing another stir-fry, quite different from the first, using some of the vegetables we had seen at the market, but did not know. Before she served us, she explained each vegetable and in which each part of Baguio it had been grown and somehow, just knowing where the vegetables had come from, made them seem even tastier and I could almost feel the goodness flowing into me

The group had bonded well by now, after all, we had shared much intimate knowledge of each other, and we sat chatting easily, having a little bit of group history to fall back on which naturally led us to sharing more about our own lives. Maria had come through with the mugs and the usual after meal coffee when a man waked off the street into the café; He seemed to be looking for somebody.

Chapter 17

The Oven

Although speaking in Filipino, we were able to understand the gist of what he was saying. "Anybody here called Maria?" he called out to the table, with a piece of paper in his hand.

"Oh, yes" Maria answered.

I looked at Maria, and then to Ellen and Greg, who were trying to look disinterested but were keen to see Maria's reaction.

"I have a delivery for you", the man continued, "an oven. Where do you want it?"

Maria spoke to the man "Hindi, hindi, no, no, there must be some mistake, I have not ordered an oven."

"Well, I have one for you, where do you want it?" he asked again.

Maria looked confused, at which point, Ellen said "It' okay Maria, it is for you. Greg and I bought it for you yesterday as we thought you could use a new oven, so tell the man where he can put it and then we can get it working".

Maria's expression changed from deep confusion, to sheer happiness and joy, and then to one of total disbelief. "Are you sure, really, did you really buy this for me Ellen?" she asked, as though she couldn't believe that she deserved such a generous gift.

"Yes, Maria, it is for you. Now would you please tell the man where to put it" Ellen said turning to Greg for his input.

"It is definitely for you. Thank you for looking after us so well" responded Greg to Ellen's expression.

"Well, in that case" she said, turning towards the man waiting slightly impatiently in the doorway, "the only place it can go is over there against the back wall". She pointed to the back of the café. I couldn't quite see how that was going to fit, but then I looked at everything else in the room, and realised that it wasn't going to create a problem at all.

The man lowered the back of his lorry, positioned a hand-truck in place, and manoeuvred the oven onto it, backed away from the lorry, turned and pushed the hand-truck into the cafe between the bar and the table and chairs and placed it at the back of the room.

"Sign here?" he said to Maria, and climbed back into his lorry and drove off.

The oven needed to be fired with propane gas. Roger disappeared downstairs somewhere and reappeared with a bottle, and connected it to the oven. Meanwhile, Maria and Ellen, together, pulled away the packaging.

"Now you are connected", Andrew said, "you need to test it to make sure that it works properly, and that the temperature is good and that it will cook evenly. The best way to do that, I would think, is to bake some cakes, just to try it out. Do you have a recipe you have used often to test it with?"

"Hmmm, well yes I do, but I am not sure that it would be a good enough recipe to try."

"I have a very well tried and tested recipe we could have a go with if you would like to try it? We could do it together". Before Maria could respond, he continued "What we will need is some self-raising flour, butter, eggs and sugar. Let's turn the oven on to get it up to temperature. Shall I come and help you with the ingredients?"

"No" Maria responded "it won't take me a minute, I'll go and collect what we need and together and we can mx it up here on the table. What should we bake it in, what type of tin?" she continued.

"The recipe is designed to make a dozen individual fairy cakes, so a tin like that would be useful".

Maria soon returned, with arms full of ingredients and the tin, some scales and a fork to mix with. Andrew had turned on the oven, and played with it for a while, to make sure he was using the correct programme, and eventually settled on one that he thought would be the best. Together, they measured out the ingredients, mixed them together, and filled the little fairy cake tin, and put it in the oven.

The pair of them, with self-satisfied expressions on their faces, pulled up a couple of chairs, and sat and watched until they were agreed and happy that the colour looked good. They pulled down the oven door, felt the top of one fairy cakes with a finger and decided they were ready for eating.

Like a couple of children, they couldn't wait for the cakes to cool down, and with a knife, loosened the edges and lifted out a cake each. "Well, I think they worked well", Maria said "Yes, the oven seems to be good" and lifted all the other cakes onto a plate and offered them around to the rest of us who had been amused by all the activity. Too full from lunch, we said we would like to try them later.

Enthused by her new piece of equipment, she thought she would like to teach us how to cook one of her dinner recipes, if we were keen to learn. Oh, yes, we definitely were, and so, again, Maria disappeared and returned with armfuls of ingredients to make a special guisado, similar to another stir-fry.

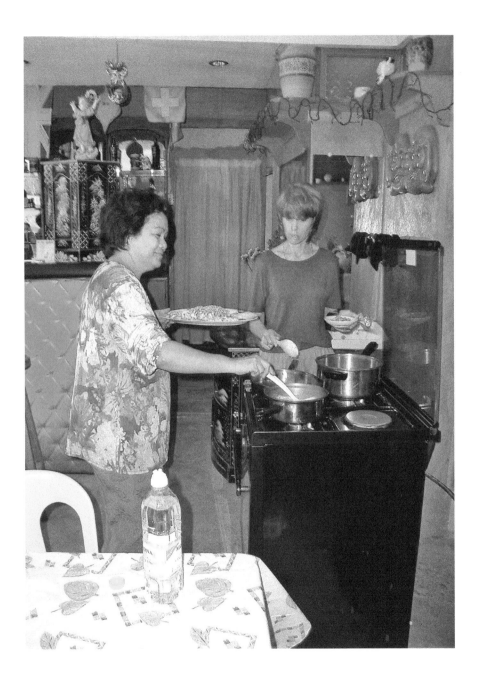

We peeled, sliced and diced tomatoes, garlic, salt, sweet peas, onion and potato, and gradually, in the correct order Maria slowly began adding ingredients and we were under strict instructions on how to stir, the correct speed with regular intervals of stopping. Ellen was there with her video camera and decided that she would film the proceedings as if it were a cookery demonstration on television. That caused much giggling and laughter. Maria had problems gauging the correct heat on the hob. The vegetables were sticking to the edge of the wok, steam should not have been rising from the liquid, and a kind of chaos and amusement ensued, attracting passers-by to pop their heads into the café to see what was going on.

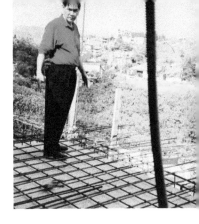

Chapter 18

New Surgery

Amidst all the capers going on in the café, Roger had been called outside to the back of his home where a large extension was being built at the rear of the property, behind his little surgery and the café.

Paul could hear Roger talking and followed the sound downwards. We all followed. At the bottom of a steep flight of steps, the footings had been dug for the extension and the slab had been laid, just, and it was still wet. Rusty metal rods had been embedded into the concrete and were flailing around in the breeze.

And then as one we all simply stared in awe at the beauty over the mountains. In the farthest distance, mountains were shrouded in a hazy mist which blended with the sky, and it was difficult to tell where one finished and the other began. Right in the centre was the airstrip on which we had landed. Surrounding it was the green valley of the steep mountainside, very lush with pine trees and mangoes. Red and green roofed houses and apartments were dotted together in clusters, settled into the landscape. Less stable, flimsy, wooden homes were embedded into tiny spots, wherever they could be built. Old motor bikes and propane gas bottles were propped against the walls of some properties. A number of them were encased in scaffolding, for the new extensions being built and this was an indication that the area was on the up with better lifestyles to look forward to.

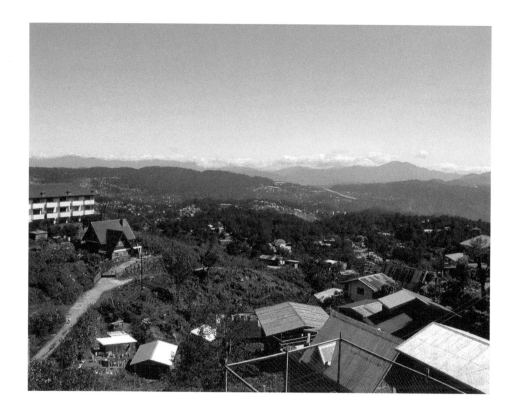

A few levels down the mountain-side clung a small community of shanty homes with a patchwork of painted corrugated tin roofs. Each tiny home had gardens created in tiers and planted with an abundance of shrubs and fruits and vegetables. It was probably easier to actually grow crops than keep trudging up and down the mountainside for food, if private transport was an issue and there seemed nowhere to keep a car, and no access either. Foot seemed to be the only way.

"The cement is still wet" Paul said, and with a glint in his eye to Roger, "Shall we leave our calling card?" and pretended to place his hand on the cement and leave an imprint of his hand.

"Yes, what a great idea! All of you do it and put your names above" he called back. "I love the idea of you all leaving your mark in the property, even though it will be covered. But you will be leaving your energy here, and I like the thought of that". And so, in playful mood we each watched each other make our imprint in the cement and write our name.

"And what are you building here?" I asked. "What will it be used for?"

"This is going to be my new operating room" Roger announced proudly." The one I am using isn't large enough and needs to be away from the café. I am getting so many more patients from around the world now, I need to expand my space and make it look a little more professional".

It was true, Paul had been investigating different psychic surgeons who were able to operate in this area of The Philippines, and had resonated well with Roger and liked the way he operated. As a consequence, Paul was bringing more and more people to him, and things had become a little tight in terms of space and also on the domestic home front. Because Paul was bringing more people, he was generating sufficient money to fund this project.

"Come", said Roger, "let me show you what I have already had built".

Winding behind him down the steep steps, he led us to a small, newly built single storey building, a one bedroom bungalow with a minute kitchenette, and a double bedroom with en-suite bathroom. It smelled of fresh paint, and had a large window, festooned in more white net. Roger was proud. "I have had this built for guests to stay in", he explained. "Some of my patients need a lot of operations and they are not always well enough to travel back and forth from a hotel, so they will be able to stay here".

I was puzzled. "Roger, if patients aren't well enough to travel back and forth from a hotel, how are they going to climb up and down these steps every time you need to operate? It is a long way to climb up?"

"They will manage", he said, "or I will operate here if I have to".

"Come on, back up to the café, we have some more operations to do. Let's get back to the surgery".

One by one, we were back on the table, and Roger did some more of the interventions he had performed in the morning, all mainly removing blockages from intestines or, in my case, some more pieces from my fibroid and ovarian cyst. Two more hours passed.

"We could sit out there", said Roger pointing down the steps again. Within a couple of minutes, he was back in the sun, with table, chairs, orange tablecloth and red and white sunshade. "Sit and make yourself comfortable, rest, you need to rest, and I will organise for us to have tea here. This will be the first time we have done this out here", he said, looking quietly satisfied with himself.

We cautiously descended down to the decking beside the concrete slab, by then almost completely dry. The sun was shining and it was beginning to feel a little warmer than it had previously been. The clouds had blown away. Roger gave Maria a hand down with the tea, and the remainder of the cakes she and Andrew had baked. Life was feeling pretty okay.

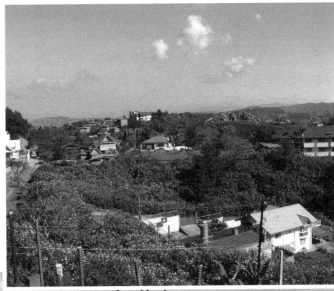

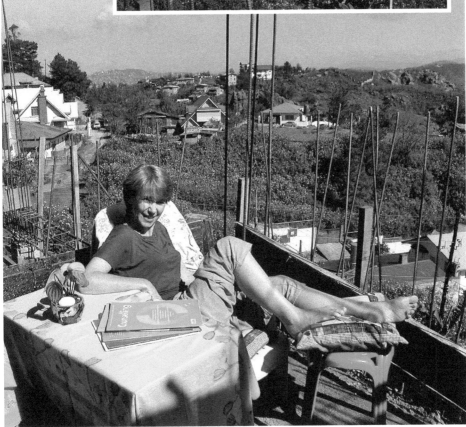

CHAPTER 19

When I am nudged by Spirit

A routine seemed to have developed within the group, even though we had only been in Baguio for three or four days. Each day began with us all gathering in the foyer of the hotel. Roger would come and collect us and we would enjoy the daily journey to Green Valley. One morning, Andrew asked Maria what was the correct way to cut a mango, and Roger stood up and instructed us all on exactly how a mango should be cut, sliced and served in typical hedgehog fashion then held it high in the air on the end of a knife. We all had to copy his example to be sure we could master this technique, much to his amusement.

After breakfast and coffee, surgery was always next on the agenda, and the reason we were there, of course. But there would always be "that" wait. Sometimes it was longer than others and one of us would ask how long we would have to wait. The answer was always the same "until the energy is ready" and sometimes adding "when I am nudged by spirit". When the time was right, and only then, Roger would spring into action to get one of us into the surgery and up on the table, always with a sense of urgency, and sometimes a little impatience. For Roger to hold the energy of spirit, and for spirit to be able to stay in the vortex was not sustainable for any great length of time, and therefore we had to take our chances as and when they became available.

"Roger", said Hannah on our fourth day there, "what do you think is stopping us from having a baby, from me conceiving?

We have tried and tried. Please see if there is anything more you can do. You have cleaned Andrew's prostate, and pulled out all sort of clots and lumpy pieces, is that enough? Is there anything actually blocking me? Can you see or do anything, please?

Roger, well aware of their situation, could only ask spirit to guide him. Hannah was up on the table.

He started scanning her body. We all assumed that he would be drawn to her uterus and fallopian tubes, but he asked her to turn over onto her stomach, and undid her bra. His hands hovered for just a second or two, and he gently pushed between her shoulder blades and his forefinger was in. With the finger and thumb of his left hand, he began pulling out clot after clot together with matter which resembled pieces of stewing steak. He laid them on her back, withdrawing his finger from the opening, wiping her with a damp cloth, leaving no scar. He scraped the pieces and the clots up into a tissue, showed Hannah what had been there and threw it all in the bin. She was dumbfounded for a moment.

"Turn over Hannah" Roger said with an intense look on his face. He placed a white towel across her stomach, and white towel over her neck, and soon his finger was piercing the base of the side of her neck and pulling out more and more blood clots and steak-like pieces of matter. Hannah instinctively closed her eyes. Roger's arms were covering her face making it difficult to focus. He withdrew his finger, and moved to her throat, and in a moment, his finger created another opening and he was pulling out more large pieces of matter and piled them up on her chest.

"Look", he said, holding up some of the pieces he had pulled away.

"What is all that?" Hannah questioned him, with a quizzical look.

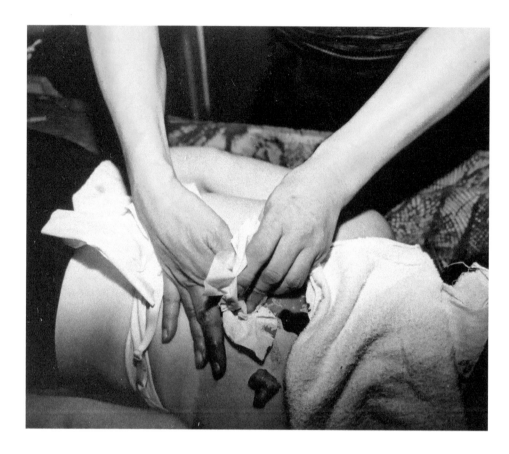

"I expect it's the result of the accident you mentioned, and a combination of a build-up of tissue and matter and emotional blockages which needs to be dealt with. You need to sit with it for a while and see if anything springs to mind about the connection of something blocking you in the mental body, and whether you can bring some clarity to the situation".

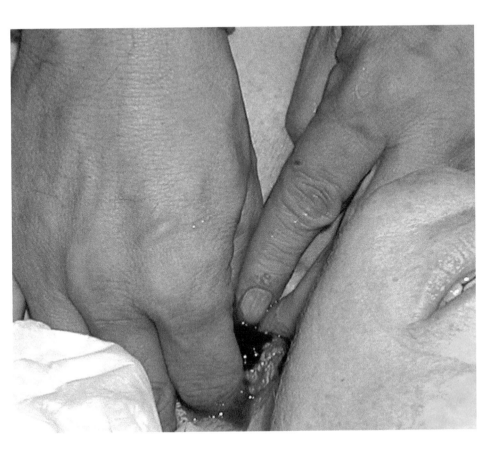

Hannah looked at him and thought, to see if anything obvious would spring to mind, but she shrugged her shoulders and said she couldn't think of anything in particular. Roger withdrew his finger, wiped the neck, leaving no mark.

He moved quickly to the other end of her body, straight to her big toe, pressed with his finger and released a vast amount of mustard coloured pus. Where there had been space in that toe was bewildering. It was as large as the toe. Roger carefully wiped it clean and for some reason, applied a pink plaster.

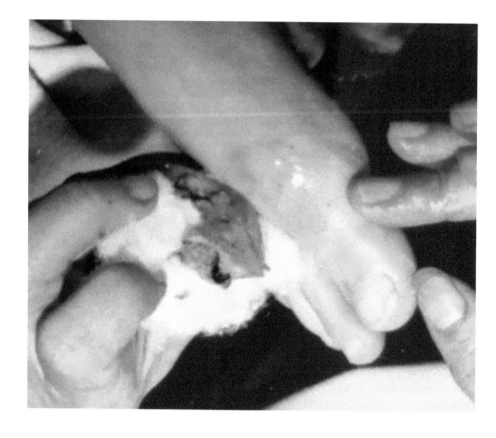

"I will leave you to lay here. Would some of you give some healing? I will be back". Andrew and Paul did just that; Paul laid his hands on her neck whilst Andrew hummed to his wife.

"Andrew, you're next, come on", Roger said impatiently. He was obviously being nudged to get on with it, and he didn't want to miss the opportunity. Andrew sat on the table and lay down and lowered his underpants a little and tee shirt up. He had a scar and had never been completely satisfied with the surgery he had received and had a feeling of discomfort in that area. Roger scanned just above the pubic bone then soon penetrated the flesh and with his forefinger and thumb pulled out a length of something gristle-like and laid it on his stomach, and then some deep red blood clots. Just a couple of inches away, Roger penetrated the flesh and pulled out more blood clots, withdrew his finger and cleaned the body. Roger had gathered together all the matter with a tissue and he picked out a length of gristle and held it up so that Andrew could see it very clearly. "This is a result of your diet. Your gut is not dealing with the food you are eating" he explained.

"A rest for you Andrew, you need to heal. I have done a lot of work. I think you are both now in a better space to make babies. This afternoon, you two are to go back to the hotel to be alone, without disturbance from others. I will keep them here and you can all meet up this evening".

For the rest of the morning, we all were up on the table, having our various operations. Paul was having small tumours removed from his liver, Ellen was having clots and blockages cleared from her intestine, I had more pieces of my fibroid pulled away and Greg had some matter removed from his shoulder. After we had all rested and lunched, Andrew and Hannah went back to the hotel for the afternoon.

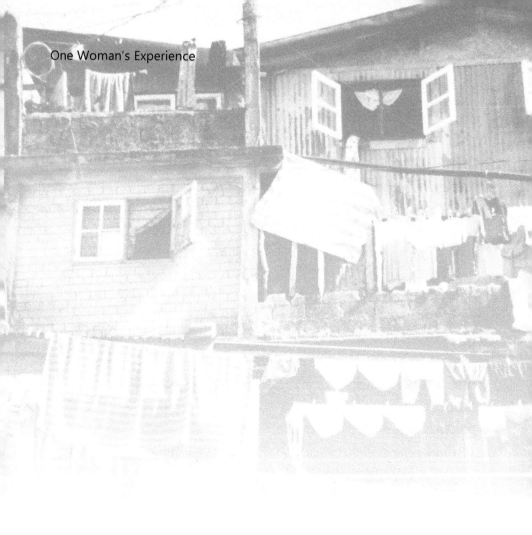

Chapter 20

An Afternoon without the Baby Makers

The rest of us sat around the table chatting and checking out the video footage Ellen and Greg had taken during the past few days. This was an interesting and a useful time as Roger was able to explain more about the surgery and how he was drawn to certain parts of the body, and more about the parts he removed.

The builders called him away to discuss the work they were doing at the back of the building, and I stretched my legs by taking a wander along the road. I spotted three of the girls from the school bus, maybe seven or eight years old. They were sat on some concrete steps, one above the other, one friend checking the other's hair for nits, chatting nineteen to the dozen. I watched briefly.

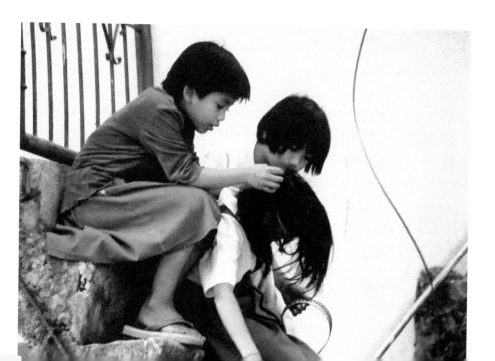

But as I slowly returned to the café, I was beginning to feel severe pains in my gut, pains of wind which had become trapped. I tried walking faster to help shift any blockage but that did not seem to help. Paul, when he saw me, asked what was wrong and I explained. Being a Reiki master, he sat down on a chair and pulled me onto his lap and put each of his hands on my stomach and back, and allowed the universal energy to flow through him and into me. I began to feel a warmth from his hands, and the pain decreased slightly, but I was too uncomfortable to be able to sit for long. I paced the room until Roger returned.

"Roger". He turned and looked at me enquiringly and could see I was in pain. "Roger, I think it must be the change of diet since I have been here, consisting mainly of fruit and vegetables, and now I have this terrible trapped wind. Could you release it or something please?"

"Hmmm", he replied, "okay", and disappeared again. Paul and I looked at each other, and he gave me some more Reiki, which helped, but I just couldn't continue to sit there, and paced some more. Roger again walked into the café.

"Roger, I am in so much pain, please, do you think you could do something, please?" I urged again.

"Yes, I will, but we have to wait".

Minutes later he suddenly said "Okay, let's go, come on, get onto the table". As I did so, I pushed my trousers down sufficiently and watched Rogers face as he scanned my abdomen. The pain increased slightly. I knew he had made an opening into my gut, when he suddenly lurched backwards, trying to avoid the bolt of wind as it released like a bullet into the air. His face screwed into a grimace. The smell was truly fowl. The others jumped backwards intuitively and then burst out laughing as they saw the comedy of it all. It worked and my pain dispersed into thin air.

Whilst I was still on the table, Roger delved deeply into my pelvis and removed several large pieces and clots which had been attached, and placed them on my stomach. Paul took several shots, getting in really close to the action as he wanted to prove in a photograph the finger just as it was about to penetrate, the depth of penetration and the fingers used to withdraw matter proving there were no scars or marks on the skin. He continued taking photos when Roger extracted more from my cyst and added them to those already on my body. All were examined closely to be sure all was healthy tissue before being tossed into the bin.

"How much is left of the fibroid, and how much of the cyst? Surely the cyst should be almost gone by now seeing that it is so much smaller than the fibroid?"

Roger picked up my right hand, and turned my palm towards him, and studied it for a while. Surprised, as I had not been aware that he had studied palmistry, I asked him "What can you see, Roger?"

"I was just checking your general health, and life lines in a different way, and I was contemplating the same question you were thinking and realising that time was running out" Roger responded. "How many more sessions and procedures would be needed, and I don't think we will have it all removed in the time that you are here. You will have to stay on, I think, for an extra two days if we are lucky".

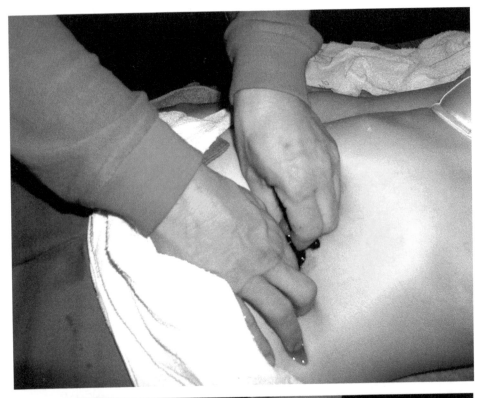

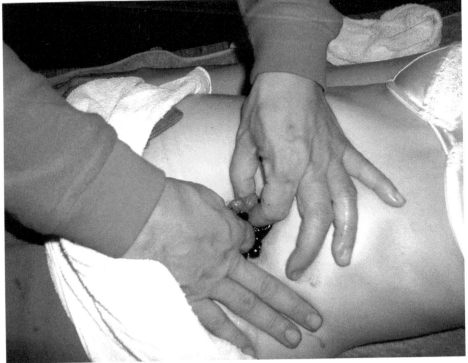

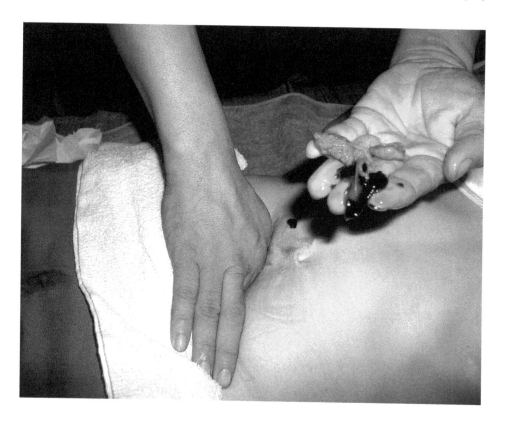

Roger delving deeply into my pelvis to remove
several large pieces and clots.

I looked at Paul who had organised the trip, and he said "We can arrange for you to change your flight back home, and we can check with the hotel to see if we can stay another two days, and then see if we can delay our stay at South China Sea Resort. This could work well, as hopefully you can return on the same flight as Hannah and Andrew and that will be better for you because you are going to need somebody to carry your suitcase as you must not lift anything heavy for a few days yet. When we get back to the hotel we will sort it out. It would be silly to return home without the job being done properly".

I was feeling conflicted. I was enjoying the most magical experience beyond my imagination up there in the mountains, in the third world, with a mouse running round, little personal hygiene, being involved in dozens of major surgical operations, without pain or scar and it had all become so natural, so normal that it had now become a way of life. On the other hand, of course, I was away from home, from my family, aware that they were trying to get on with life and not only was Laura no longer with us, I was not there with them either. I knew it was not easy.

"This is so much better than before" Roger said to Paul as he pulled more tumours from his liver. "Your diet is serving you well and cutting out the fish and particularly sushi, has really helped".

"I agree, at least none of these are cancerous, as were all the others you have removed in the past, but I also think the coffee enemas have helped". Paul had not only dramatically changed his diet a couple of years earlier, but he routinely, each morning, gave himself a coffee enema to cleanse the liver, which seemed to be having a very positive effect. Certainly it had been some months since there was any sign of cancer as he continued the habit.

Paul, Greg and I took it in turns to stand on the chair to get an overhead vantage point of Ellen's operations. Roger had pulled several lengths of matter similar to gristle, from the bends of her intestines which had been causing her great discomfort. Greg was low to her abdomen, recording these precise moments and the explanation and description of the pieces as Roger examined them. It was important that these recordings had real clarity and authenticity. To the rest of the world, what was happening would not be normal.

It was the end of the afternoon by the time we had all had, or helped with, our various operations and the healing periods in between. Over a cup of tea we chatted about the day's events and the fact that I would be staying longer and return with Hannah and Andrew whilst Greg and Ellen would be leaving on a different flight to extend their time away from. Paul would be staying in the Philippines for an extra time. So, earlier than had become usual, Roger drove us back to the hotel so that we could re-arrange my flight booking before we all went to a restaurant for dinner.

Chapter 21

Seeing is Believing

Next morning, Roger had collected us all and driven us back to the café for breakfast. We had finished our coffee and unusually, Roger was raring to go and called us all in to the surgery. "Right Greg, your turn".

No sooner was Greg up on the table, than Roger was already scanning, and went directly to Greg's face. "Okay, did you know you had a problem with your eyes? You have a cataract, but hold on, and I will show you" he said almost under his breath". And with that he held the eyelids apart with his forefinger and thumb of his left hand, and with the pad of his right forefinger, just wiped the pupil with a downward motion and the cataract came away on his finger. "Pass me that glass over there and a cotton bud please," he said, and then wiped the cataract from his finger with the cotton bud and placed the cataract onto the glass for us all to see. It had all been done in seconds. I looked at Greg to see how he was and he was staring at everything in a new way as his vision was now much clearer. Roger had made this seem so simple and to this day, I wonder why we can't all do that, and why in western medicine it is so much more complicated?

"Okay, before you rest, I need to look at the side of your head" Roger was saying. Greg turned as he was directed to do. Roger leant towards the table beside him and picked up a cocktail stick, turned to Greg and almost immediately felt behind his ear and gently pushed the stick into his skull, with as much ease as if he was just pushing it through some putty. Out came some fleshy matter and a clot, and after closing the opening, studied the pieces and satisfied they were healthy, threw them into the bin. He disappeared and returned with another spring onion with both ends removed, and placed it in Greg's ear. "Leave it there for a quarter of an hour whilst you heal. I will be back." Ellen stood with her hands on her husband's body, sending him some healing.

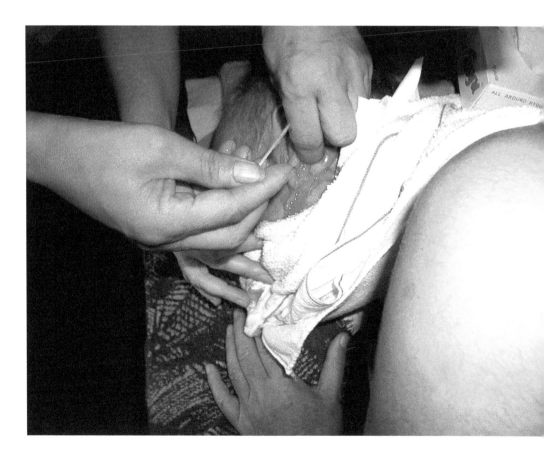

Whilst I stood witnessing the situation I heard Andrew say "Roger, do you know where there is a Barber? I need to get my hair cut".

"Yes, I do. I can do it for you" he replied.

None of us were sure that we had heard correctly and Andrew said "Did you say you could do it?

Almost before he had finished his sentence, Roger had pulled out a bag of brushes and combs, scissors and a black towel and, pointing to a chair, showed Andrew that he wanted him to sit there, then wrapped a towel around him and pushed his head forward. Very confidently, he sprayed the hair with water from a spray bottle and started cutting. Notoriously, wavy hair can be difficult to style but the end result left Andrew beaming and amused.

"That looks great Roger" said Hannah, and cheekily added "would you mind doing mine too please?" She and Andrew had similar hair.

"Yes, of course, come on" and wrapped a towel around her shoulders as she sat down. This seemed surreal to all of us, and it was a little difficult to absorb. I had to keep re-assessing my reality. There we were up in the mountains, having psychic bare-hand surgery, with a mouse having been running round the room, not too sure about the hygiene, and in between operations, the surgeon was cutting hair. Strangely bizarre, but real, and Roger sprayed and cut her hair and allowed it to dry naturally. Hannah was thrilled.

The days continued their rhythm until the final day came. Roger had collected not just us, but also our suitcases. The breakfast table was set, and we all gathered and sat down and ate. As coffee was being finished, and the conversation had become a touch sad at our leaving, Ellen, pulled a large carrier bag from beside her chair, took out a tall plant, an orchid. Ellen stood up and carried it over to Maria and handed it to her to say "thank you for everything" and that she and Greg appreciated the hospitality they had received. Maria beamed her own thanks back and gave it pride of place up on the alter table.

"Okay" said Roger, "We still have work to do, come on, I am ready right now".

I was still loving my time there and happy that it was not quite all over yet. I still had time to treasure another hour or two with this very special, very ordinary, very humbling man.

What I didn't know was that Ellen was going to have an operation I had not seen Roger perform before. This was the only one where I was holding my breath, as I watched. "Ellen, you have a blockage of some sort in your sinuses, close to the bridge of your nose. It might be a little uncomfortable for you, but just remember to keep breathing. It is important that I do this. Keep breathing."

Roger covered her eyes with a white towel so that she couldn't see what he was doing. He took two cocktail sticks and pushed them up each nostril. He knew exactly what he was doing, but it looked very painful. Ellen was obviously feeling uncomfortable and instinctively was pushing her head backwards, away from the pressure.

"Keep breathing, almost done" Roger said, trying to keep her calm.

"There", he said, "all finished. Look," he said, uncovering her eyes, pulled a tissue from the box and picked up the matter he had withdrawn. "Now you will find that you can breathe more easily, and everything else will feel better too. You may even think with more clarity".

Ellen looked at the tissue, and then at Roger and said "that was really uncomfortable, and although it didn't really hurt, I was anticipating that it would, but I am so grateful to not have that in me anymore. Gosh, thank you so much, thank you".

For me, Roger had removed the last piece of cyst the day before, and now took out the last of the fibroid. I felt so pleased and happy and grateful to Roger, but there seemed no way to voice my gratitude sufficiently. It was impossible, and he well understood that.

With more hugs and goodbyes, Greg and Ellen climbed into a taxi to holiday for a few more days, elsewhere in the world. It was all arranged. The men packed Roger's vehicle with our luggage and we all said our final farewells to him with commitments of keeping in contact, with him and each other. We all piled into the vehicle with Maria in the driver's seat and waved goodbye to Roger, and the café, and Green Valley.

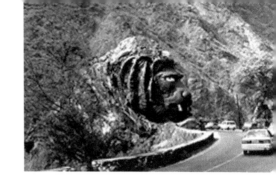

CHAPTER 22

The Lion's Head

Our trip to The Philippines was not yet over, although our visit to Baguio was. Paul had booked us into the South China Sea Resort for a couple of nights, a westward drive of about an hour and a half. Leaving the height of the mountain behind, and heading for the sea, would always be a downhill and beautifully scenic journey. Kennon Road was long and slowly we began our descent as it weaved us around sharp bends showing fleeting glimpses of the mountain tops surrounding us, and the valley below.

After some seriously zig-zagging bends, there in an isolated area half way through our journey, an amazing and unexpected structure towered at the edge of the road. The largest sculpture, a massive iconic lions head had been carved from a limestone boulder of the mountain. Maria had kept this truly unexpected surprise quietly to herself, and happily obliged when we insisted on stopping for this astonishing photo opportunity. When standing next to the Lion itself, we barely came up to its mouth. Maria explained that this incredibly impressive piece of artwork was completed in 1973 and commissioned by The Lions Club.

We set off again for the lowlands of La Union, and the beach to rest and recuperate. I was looking forward to some time to do absolutely nothing, to just laze on the beach and take in some sun.

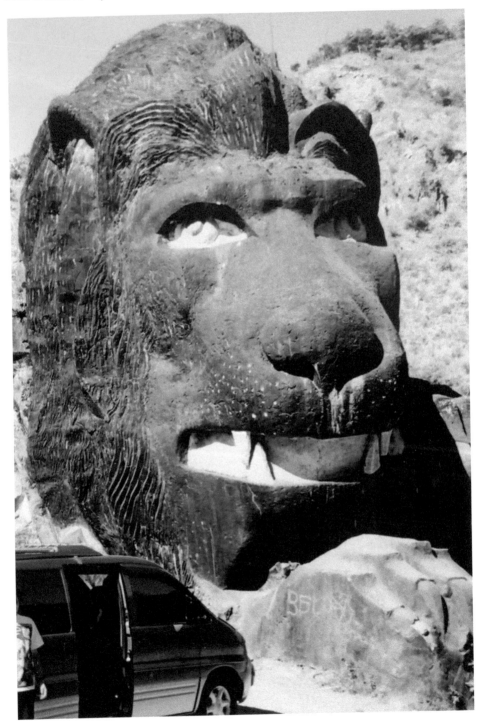

Chapter 23

The Resort

It was late afternoon when our suitcases were unloaded. The temperature here was much hotter than up in Baguio, and I was keen to change into something cooler. We all checked in and found our way to our rooms, set out in the grassy grounds margined with palm trees. Paul carried my case for me, as I was under strict instructions from Roger that I was not allowed to lift anything heavy for a few days.

My room was clean, painted white with pale ceramic tiled floor, and with an en-suite bathroom. It was very simple yet had a certain charm about it. White fluffy towels had been twisted and folded into swans on the bed, and a typical Filipino painting hung on a wall. Quickly, I changed into light clothing.

We had not yet said our farewells to Maria whom we had invited to stay for some refreshment after our journey. She had gone ahead and was waiting for us in the bar and I soon found her sipping a large glass of papaya juice.

Sitting almost on the beach, the bar was a tall structure having a roof loosely thatched with long reeds and grasses. The internal wooden structure was beautifully engineered creating an architectural statement. Three walls were little more than window spaces fitted with bamboo roller blinds to give some protection from storms. I crossed to a table by the 'window' and joined Maria. She was staring out to sea, in a private world of her own. I sensed she would have loved to have stayed here with us for a couple of days, and enjoy some much needed rest. As it was, she stayed just a short time, and was soon heading back to her home, her children and Roger. We were saddened to say goodbye.

Having not eaten for a few hours, we enjoyed toasties and cool drinks in the shade of a palm tree as we absorbed the atmosphere and the views. Between low stone walls which separated the hotel from the narrow beach, a couple of long stone steps reached down onto the dark sand which was rather solid and muddy looking. It formed part of a bay, where the mountain dipped its toes into the sea, here and there, and then gave way to more sandy beaches margined with palm trees which separated the beaches from the lowland.

School was out, and children were playing on the beach, holding a few sweets in their hands, chatting away. Some of the boys used the safe space to ride their bicycles and taking home shopping from the local supermarket as younger brothers and sisters ran alongside them. Another girl, a budding photographer, stood taking some shots of the coastline and sun as it began to lower on the skyline.

Far out on the horizon, a flotilla of boats, mere specs in the distance very gradually drew closer and their slim and brightly coloured yellow, blue and red hulls became more visible. The pulse of the oarsmen was steady as they were heading for shore, towards us.

It wasn't long before crowds on the shoreline had gathered and families with young children all clambered forward. The rowing stopped and men at the bows of the boats threw lines to those ashore. Individuals grabbed them and with the help of others, began the arduous task of pulling the boats from the deeper to more shallow water.

The crews then jumped overboard and stood waist high in the sea. With a sequence much practiced, they lifted the boats by their long wooden floats which were attached to the sides, and eased them high up onto their shoulders. People on the shore, dashed into the water, and as unified teams, together carried the boats beyond the tide line and onto stands set into the beach. As the women and children took over, unloading the catch of the day, the men washed down each boat making sure it would be in good order and ready for duty the following day.

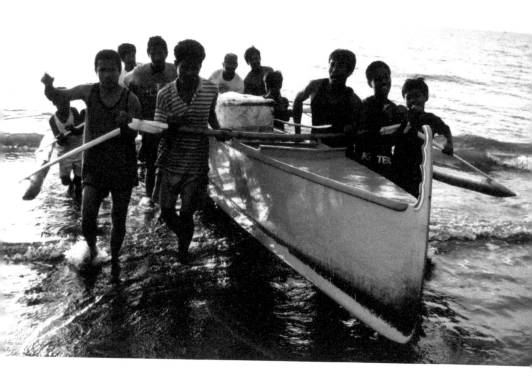

Further along where the beach, and extending back towards the road, shabby white concrete block buildings and scruffy wooden sheds with corrugated tin roofs had been cobbled together to store crates, nets and oars. Beside them, canopies made from a hotchpotch of timber and thatch sheltered the women as they sorted the days catch into plastic crates for markets, or prepared fish for their own suppers.

We walked along the beach, in and amongst the crowds, with our cameras, recording real local life. The natives were very happy for us to photograph them. The mood was buoyant and festive. One of the older fishermen, who called himself Armando, tried explaining to us the methods they used to catch fish. Roberto was repairing and cleaning his nets in readiness for the following days catch. One of the younger boys, aged about twelve, Toto, showed us the bait he used for line fishing; fish made of a metal, one painted blue and one red with white undersides and black eyes. These would be hung over the side of the boat in the hope that something would bite.

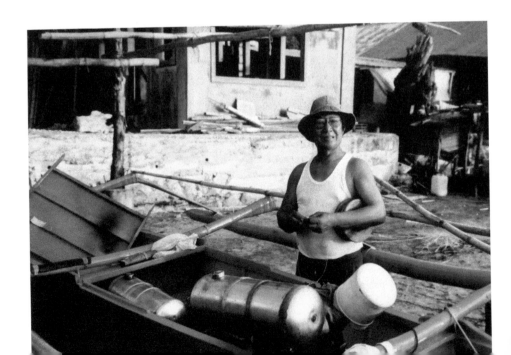

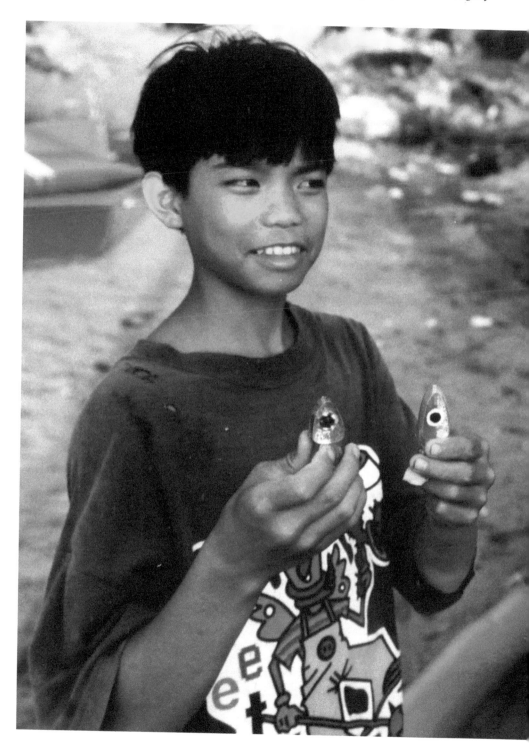

I felt we were made to feel so welcome, when one particular lady and her children urged us to stay and eat with them, but we could see that they really had barely enough to feed themselves, and it was too late to take something to contribute, so we sadly and appreciatively declined their very generous offer.

The light faded in simply a matter of minutes, and we watched as the sky turned a golden streaky glow, lighting and colouring the sea as it dipped below the horizon. Behind us, the lights of the fires glowed and the parents and children grouped together on the sand, eating as one.

The following morning, I awoke to the sound of gulls calling overhead. There was some urgency to their calls. I lifted my head from the pillow and took the robe still lying on the bed and pulled it around me. Unlocking and opening the door, I stepped outside and tiptoed in bare feet over to the white concrete posts and painted rails separating me from the beach. The gulls were fighting over the remains of fish from the night before, and were dragging the carcasses along the shore line. The warmth of the early morning sun felt good on my skin. I showered, put on my bathing costume under a casual dress, ready for the day ahead.

I was first at breakfast, and started without them. I studied the menu in great detail. It was good to have the time to quietly consider what I would like and mull over the options of how I might spend the day. I could swim in the pool, or in the sea. I could walk to the next village along the beach, or maybe there was some water activity I had yet to discover?

The waiter came across to my table. He had a great energy about him, happy and smiling. I ordered mango and papaya, toast and coffee. Waiting for my food to arrive, I poured a glass of water, and sipped it and stared out across the bay. My thoughts were interrupted by the waiter bringing my breakfast on a large tray.

"Here you are madam, the coffee is very hot, be careful", he said as he laid everything in front of me.

"Do you have anything planned for the day? he asked.

"Nothing that I have decided upon", I answered, "Maybe I will just wait and see how the day pans out".

"Enjoy your breakfast", he said, and I smiled my thanks to him.

Settling back into my thoughts, I was soon brought back to the current moment, when Hannah and Andrew pulled out chairs facing me, sat down and beckoned to the waiter for the menu. They were about to order when Paul joined us and placed his order. He had been here many times before and knew exactly what he would be having.

Totally relaxed, we found endless things to talk about, particularly from the past two weeks. What we hadn't known was that Paul had planned a talk about diet, nutrition and emotional energy. He had booked a small room for us all and when eventually we moved away from breakfast, we followed him. He explained to us in more detail than Roger had, the importance of a macrobiotic diet, and only eating food grown locally and in season, avoiding sugar and wheat, fish, meat and dairy, basically. For each of us he explained in more detail what would work best, and he was full of examples and testimonials for us to realise that we need to take heed. In somewhat less detail, Paul explained about how our emotions block our energy and that in itself was a major concern for our health.

Although we already knew of the other healing modalities he used, he went into some detail about the courses he was running and how it may be useful to us to learn some of them. Having already experienced the benefits of Reiki I was enthusiastic, and had already decided that I would take the next available course.

Those days simply lazing around at the resort was exactly what was needed. November had turned into December, and to feel the warmth of the sun, to swim a little in the warm sea, watch the local people, and chatting with those I had grown to care about, was exactly what any doctor would have ordered.

And then we were heading to Manila and the long flights to Dubai and then London. It would feel strange to leave this country behind, and all the intimate times with Roger, all being filmed, or photographed and the laughter and tears we had shed. Yes, it had been quite an emotional involvement in each other's lives. Would that continue once we were back in the U.K I wondered?

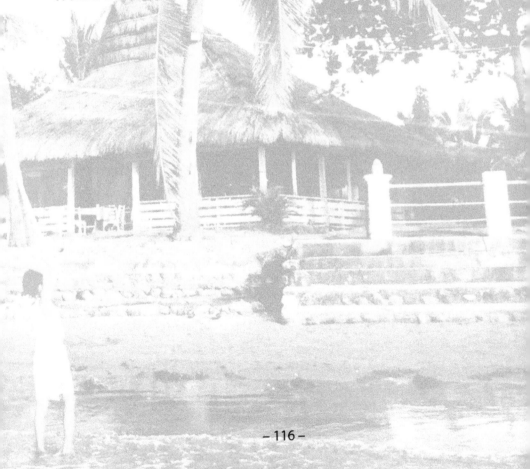

CHAPTER 24

Back Home

Settling back into being home again, I spent a few days reflecting, processing and digesting the awesomeness of that which we had all experienced. And yet, because it felt so natural to each of us, it was without "awe". We had taken the wonderness of it, the greatness of it in our stride as the most natural and innate way of healing. Trying to vocalise my experience to myself, yet alone to my husband and son, without some visual support, was not easy for them to comprehend my words. But that changed, once I had collected all the photographs I had been waiting to have developed, and their appreciation of my journey grew and they were fascinated by all that they saw. These were days before digital cameras and when film was developed into printed photographs and took time, usually days.

A week or so later Greg and Ellen invited the group to their home for a get-together so that we could share the video footage and study the photographs we had all taken. Greg and Ellen had also been looking forward to showing us their home; very fresh and contemporary, with original abstract artwork, and all carrying a wonderful energy.

Ellen had always taken an interest in food, and she and Paul had talked about food and diet during the years they had known each other prior to this particular trip. Ellen, it seemed, bought most of her groceries from the health food shop in her local village, and put on an amazing spread using foods I had not even heard of, yet alone tried. I was surprised. We enjoyed experimenting and were grateful for the opportunity.

We spent several hours reminiscing over the photos, the video footage both couples had taken, and comparing notes. It felt right that we were together and honouring our journey. It felt important.

CHAPTER 25

Showing my GP

Before my trip, I had mentioned to my doctor my plans to have my fibroid and cyst removed, not on the NHS, or even in the UK, but by a psychic bare-hand surgeon in the Philippines. He clearly had no way of understanding my reasoning, my explanation of what, without doubt, would happen, and he seemed unable to comprehend the concept, and thought I would be "opening up a whole can of worms"! He thought I was crazy, and shaking his head in disbelief, wished me good luck.

Having been back home a couple of weeks, I thought it may be interesting to call my doctor to let him know that my fibroid and my cyst had been removed, they were no longer part of me, and that I had photos and a video he was welcome to watch. He tentatively agreed to do so.

A few days later after lunch, he arrived at my home. He seemed slightly uneasy. "Maybe he thinks he has come to a coven!" I thought, slightly bemused. I switched on the video player and showed him the very clear video footage of parts of my fibroid being removed in sections. I explained that it would have been too dangerous to carry out a single operation. He could see quite easily, the imagery of the video footage was clear, Roger inserting his fingers into my abdomen, over my fibroid and pulling pieces of tissue, matter, flesh, clots and placing them on me and then explaining to me and to camera what they were. He studied the stills of the same operations, and because they were stills, exact and precise details were clearly defined.

I looked at him, waiting for some comments, or observations, something, anything! In the end I asked him "So, what do you think?" by way of making conversation.

"Well", he said, "It certainly looks as though they have been removed, and the photos do show that they look like they are being removed, and the film looks as though they have been removed, but I can't believe it. The only way I could accept that that was what happened, would be if you were totally naked, the surgeon was totally naked and that you were lying on a glass bed so that I could see that there was no trickery".

I was astounded. How could anybody be that closed, that suspicious, that fearful? What was he frightened of? Why could he not rejoice in the wonderment of it? I lay down on the carpet, perfectly flat.

"Here", I said, unzipping my trousers, "Check for yourself. You know how large the fibroid was and how misshapen it made my abdomen. Feel".

He knelt down on both knees, and placed his hand on my abdomen where the fibroid once was. He felt and he pushed down deeper and deeper, until it was actually quite painful

"So what do you think now?"

"It certainly seems to have gone, I can't feel it. For me to believe it though, you will need to have an x-ray. I will go back now to the surgery and arrange it for you".

"Sorry", I said. "There is no way I am having an x-ray. Firstly, I have nothing to prove to you, or to anybody else. I know exactly what happened. I was there, as were the other people, but I was just giving you the opportunity to see something different, and I rather thought you may be fascinated to watch those operations, and to actually have had one of your patients go all that way, and experience that. It is almost as authentic as seeing it first-hand with your own eyes. Secondly, I went all the way to The Philippines to have drug-free treatment which did not include dangerous practices like x-rays. Sorry, but there is no way I am doing that. It is not critical".

"Well", he said, "that is the only way I can be sure. It would be scientific and then I could trust what I have seen.

This was the first time I really understood that actually many doctors are frightened of truth, hiding behind the Medical Council and putting their own financial security before their patients' health.

I am not saying that all Western Medicine should be shunned. Not at all, as it can serve us well in times of emergency and when we need a quick fix. If I had an accident resulting in a broken shin bone, this would require fairly immediate attention, and the bone reset. Being bitten by a deadly venomous snake would need serum as quickly as possible. A mother about to give birth may need an emergency caesarean section as it may be too dangerous to have a vaginal delivery. There are times when western medicine is critical and appropriate.

As I said at the beginning of the book, I had rarely told my story, except with those I felt would be interested. It has not been easy for others to grasp the fact that at the time there were only three places in the world where the energy vortexes enabled such surgery to be performed. They argued that this could be done elsewhere, and without exception, each of them told me of somebody they knew who had had psychic bare-hand surgery, and would explain in great detail how it was performed. Some referred to basic energy healing that many of us can do, some referred to healers with spirit and guides entering the body, and moving energy and performing non-physical operations. Another spoke of a healer who went into an altered state who was completely taken over by spirit, whose clothes became loose and twisted and with a knife performed surgery!

None of this has the slightest semblance to the psychic bare-hand surgery and my own personal interactions and involvement with the actual surgery up in the mountains in The Philippines. There, Roger simply connected with, but was never taken over by spirit. He was always laughing with us, speaking and explaining to us everything he was extracting from us, leaving no scar or trace of any sort. He involved me in some of the surgery, and I actually helped to pull out some matter from others when an extra finger was needed during the seventy-one operations he performed between us.

For our part, as patients, we never took any anaesthetic, any pain killers, no drugs, no alcohol, never felt any pain at all, and were wide awake and interacting with everybody in the room at all times. I could describe this surgery as supernatural, because it was certainly super, and could not have been more natural. Perhaps "superbly natural" would be better.

Most people who champion "natural, organic" healing acknowledge that illness is a side-effect of negative thought patterns, toxins and diet, although not always on a conscious level and that it is important to remove the root cause of the problem, and take responsibility for our own health, enabling real and permanent healing to take place.

The whole experience of my trip to The Philippines, was a springboard to my future conscious awareness and further awakening, which I have actively encouraged its evolution. My journey before, and since, has been a huge learning curve, one that is evolving in continuum. There have been many challenges along the way; much ebb and flow needed for spiritual growth and all very necessary.

Now that you have read my story, I ask you:

"If you needed major surgery, would you consider making my journey yours?

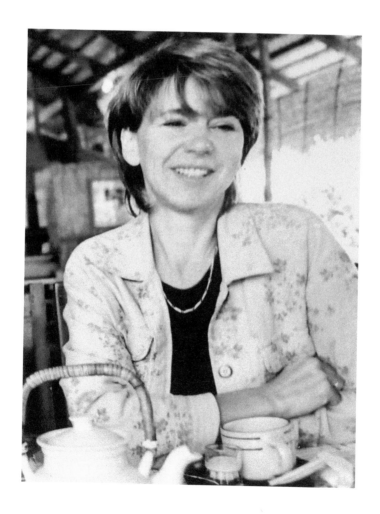

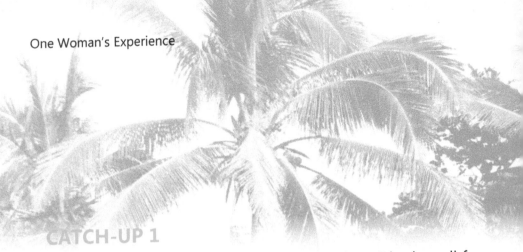

CATCH-UP 1

Not long after my return from The Philippines, I had a call from my G.P.

"A patient of mine needs surgery and she doesn't want to go along the normal channels. I mentioned to her your experience and we are wondering if you could let us have more information please! Then if she is interested, would you be prepared to talk to her about it?"

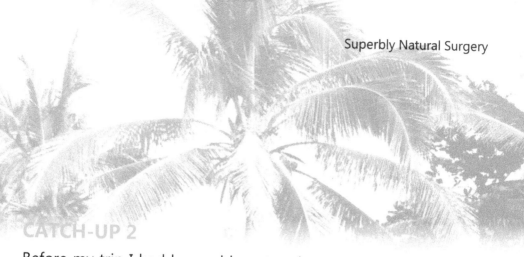

CATCH-UP 2

Before my trip I had learned how to take people into past lives and since my return I learned many differing techniques using vibration and frequency, and at one point I was channelling paintings of souls. I had a good and clear understanding of how to live in a healthy higher frequency.

So, it came as a shock to me some time after my return to find my abdomen misshapen again and could feel that the fibroid had returned, overnight it seemed. I did not understand what had happened and called my G.P. He told me something I had no idea about, that fibroids even if removed in the normal way, sometimes did regrow.

I contemplated the situation for a while then realised what had caused it to happen. I had failed to deal with core issues initially, the emotional issues which manifested into a fibroid in the first place. Back then though, I had no knowledge that emotional issues manifest into physical issues and I don't think I knew that before visiting Roger. Had I realised, had I known, I could have worked on any issues before my visit. Paul had mentioned trapped emotions when he gave us a lecture in the South China Sea Resort but it didn't really register sufficiently well with me. The emotions were still trapped within my physical body. My understanding is that fibroids are often the result of emotional issues concerning the feminine body, and motherhood and all the feelings and stresses that are catapulted onto us. There is also another very important factor, which then was barely touched upon, and that is the environment and the toxins therein which are responsible for much physical trauma.

I changed my diet to one totally alkaline with specific herbs for quite a few months and then I just seemed to forget about it. I have done much inner work, alone and with many therapists in order that I can live in a high vibration. Now, many years later, I barely give the fibroid a second thought, and quite honestly, I am not sure if it is even there. I am giving it no attention.

My experience in the Philippines was profound and changed my view of the world dramatically. I could not help but realise everything is energy and although many things are not probable they are possible. It is a matter of mind-set and being curious about life, seeking spiritual adventures and being open and not closed to experiences, open to receiving high energy, open to a different way of thinking, and listening to advice and information. Ask questions to others. Ask questions to yourself. Ask questions to source. Drop the ego and listen and watch for the answers.

I have noticed over years with people, that it is difficult for them to move forward to raise their vibration simply because they are unable to trust. Even if they have dipped their toes in the water, or even waded up to their knees on their spiritual journey, if they cannot trust then they are not committed to the process. Work needs to be done to heal the issue of trust, to move forward.

Trust, for me, is about what feels right, what feels authentic and not allowing others to infiltrate my own personal trust boundaries. If trust boundaries are over-ridden then I am not being true to myself and my vibration would not remain as high.

I hope you have found this book interesting, even fascinating, and that it encourages you to embark further on your own voyage of discovery. By raising your vibration you are raising the vibration of our planet. Our planet needs you. Go, fly!

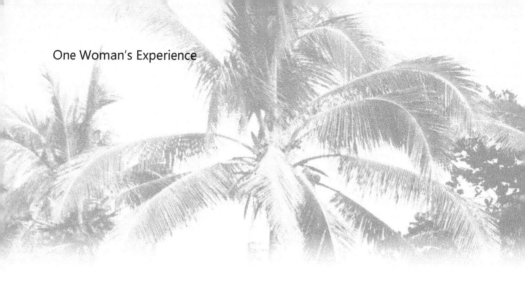

One Woman's Experience

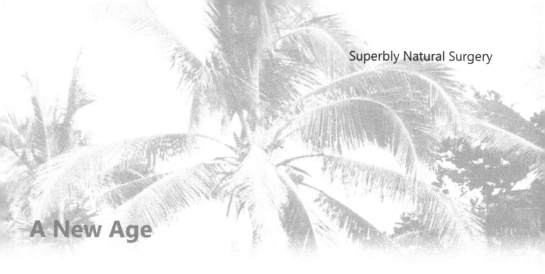

A New Age

We are now entering the new Age of Aquarius and will soon also be moving into the Golden Age. These are such exciting times and we are so lucky to have chosen this time to be here on the Earth plane. Our lives will become more spiritual and our vibration raised and we will be aware.

Listen with your ears

and with your eyes

and with your heart

Give others the time and space to tell their story